Femoral Head and Neck Anatomy and Pathology

Bahaa Medlej
Israel Hershkovitz

Femoral Head and Neck Anatomy and Pathology

Anatomy of the hip joint and its relation to lesions in the femoral head and neck

LAP LAMBERT Academic Publishing

Impressum / Imprint

Bibliografische Information der Deutschen Nationalbibliothek: Die Deutsche Nationalbibliothek verzeichnet diese Publikation in der Deutschen Nationalbibliografie; detaillierte bibliografische Daten sind im Internet über http://dnb.d-nb.de abrufbar.
Alle in diesem Buch genannten Marken und Produktnamen unterliegen warenzeichen-, marken- oder patentrechtlichem Schutz bzw. sind Warenzeichen oder eingetragene Warenzeichen der jeweiligen Inhaber. Die Wiedergabe von Marken, Produktnamen, Gebrauchsnamen, Handelsnamen, Warenbezeichnungen u.s.w. in diesem Werk berechtigt auch ohne besondere Kennzeichnung nicht zu der Annahme, dass solche Namen im Sinne der Warenzeichen- und Markenschutzgesetzgebung als frei zu betrachten wären und daher von jedermann benutzt werden dürften.

Bibliographic information published by the Deutsche Nationalbibliothek: The Deutsche Nationalbibliothek lists this publication in the Deutsche Nationalbibliografie; detailed bibliographic data are available in the Internet at http://dnb.d-nb.de.
Any brand names and product names mentioned in this book are subject to trademark, brand or patent protection and are trademarks or registered trademarks of their respective holders. The use of brand names, product names, common names, trade names, product descriptions etc. even without a particular marking in this works is in no way to be construed to mean that such names may be regarded as unrestricted in respect of trademark and brand protection legislation and could thus be used by anyone.

Coverbild / Cover image: www.ingimage.com

Verlag / Publisher:
LAP LAMBERT Academic Publishing
ist ein Imprint der / is a trademark of
AV Akademikerverlag GmbH & Co. KG
Heinrich-Böcking-Str. 6-8, 66121 Saarbrücken, Deutschland / Germany
Email: info@lap-publishing.com

Herstellung: siehe letzte Seite /
Printed at: see last page
ISBN: 978-3-659-28639-1

Zugl. / Approved by: Tel-Aviv, Tel-Aviv University, Diss., 2011

To my parents,
Omar and Rifka Medlej,
Thanks

TABLE OF CONTENTS

LIST OF FIGURES

13

LIST OF TABLES

18

LIST OF APPENDICES

PREFACE

Our sincere thanks go to Dr. Charlie Greenwald for initiating the project; to Professor Bruce Latimer and Lyman Jellema from the Cleveland Museum of Natural History, Cleveland, Ohio for making the project feasible; to Anna Behar who did all the illustrations; to the Dan David Foundation, the Tassia and Dr. Joseph Meychan Chair for the History and Philosophy of Medicine, and to Joe Shefran for their financial support. To all our colleagues in the lab: Dr. Youssef Masharawi, Dr. Gali Dar, Dr. Smadar Peleg, Dr. Nili Steinberg-Knopp, Hila May, Haim Cohen, Janan Abbas, Dr. Rachel Sarig, Dr. Tatiana Sella-Tunis, Viviane Slon, Dan Stein and Rachel Oz for their support and good company during and after the work. Mostly, to our families in Barta'a and Hod Hasharon.

1. INTRODUCTION

The head and neck of the femur manifest several lesions (i.e. Allen's fossa, Porier facet) which are unique to the hip joint. Although widely used by anthropologists as an indication of specific habitual activities (Kostick, 1963; Angel, 1964), their etiology has never been established. In addition to their anthropological significance, these lesions have important clinical significance. The purpose of the current research is firstly, to characterize the lesions anatomically and demographically and secondly, to decipher their etiology and pathophysiology (Pitt et al., 1982; Siebenrock et al., 2004; Jager et al., 2004; Leunig et al., 2005).

1.1. Anatomy of the hip joint

The aim of the following anatomical discussion is to present the main morphological features of the hip joint and its components. These features are later used to decipher the pathophysiology of several lesions on the head and the neck of the femur. The anatomical description is divided in to three sub-chapters: the acetabulum (1.1.1.1), femur head and neck (1.1.1.2) and the hip joint capsule (1.1.1.3).

1.1.1 Joint Structures

1.1.1.1 The acetabulum:

The hip is a diarthrodial ball and socket joint, linking the head of the femur with the cup-shaped fossa, or cavity, of the acetabulum (Gray, 1985) (Figures 1). The primary function of the hip joint is to support the weight of the upper body segment, in a static, erect position.

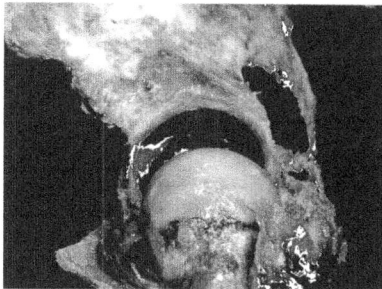

Figure 1: dissection of the hip joint notes the reception of the head of the femur into the cup-shaped cavity of the pelvis (acetabulum), lateral view; open capsule (author work).

The acetabulum is a cup-like concave socket, located slightly inferiorly, occupying the lateral aspect of the inominate (os coxa) bone. The acetabulum is composed of three bones: the pubis (1/5), the ischium (2/5), and the ileum (2/5) (Moor and Dally, 1999) (Figure 2). Full synostosisi of the three bones occurs by age 20. The acetebular cavity faces obliquely forward, outward and downward. The inferior tilt of the acetabulum (in living individuals measured as the center edge [CE] angle or the angle of Wiberg) dictates the overlap between the femoral head and the acetabulum (Figure 3). In males it approximately $38°$ and in females $35°$ (Adna et al., 1986). A smaller CE angle, produced by a more vertical orientation of the acetabulum, may result in reduced coverage of the head of the femur. As the CE angle increases with age, coverage of the head of the femur decreases, causing reduced joint stability. The anterior orientation of the acetabulum, known as the acetabular anteversion, is $18.50°$ for males and $21.50°$ for females (Kapandji, 1987). An increase in the anteversion angle results in decreased joint stability.

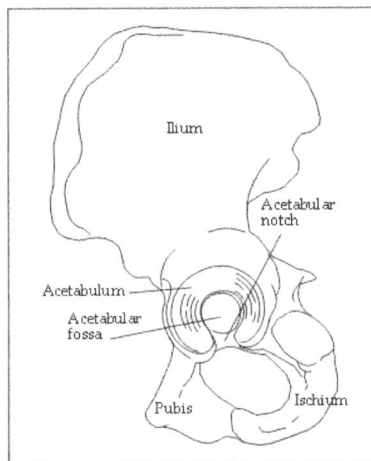

Figure 2: schematic drawing, showing the three parts of the inominate that form the acetabular fossa are the ilium, ischium, and pubis (author work).

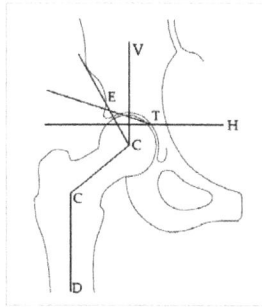

Figure 3: the center edge angle of the acetabulum is formed between a vertical line through the center of the femoral head and a line connecting the center of the femoral head and the bony edge of the acetabulum (adapted from http://www.alfigueiredo.com/sobrecobertura.html).

The acetabulum inner surface is covered by articular hyaline cartilage and is thickened on the periphery (Kempson et al., 1971; Rushfeld et al., 1979). A flat fibro cartilage band connected to the rim at the acetabulum together with the transverse ligament, called the labrum, adds depth to the acetabular socket. It's main function however, is to grasp the head of the femur, thereby maintaining contact with the acetabulum. In addition, the labrum contains nerves leading to the acetabulum (Kim and Azuma, 1995). The inner articular surface of the acetabulum, called the lunate surface, is horse-shoe shaped and covered by hyaline cartilage. The lunate surface joins with the head of the femur. The inferior position of the lunate surface is dissected by a deep notch, called the acetabular notch. The deepest, non- articulated portion of the acetabulum is called the acetabular fossa, and contains fibroelastic fat, covered with a synovial membrane. This fossa is essential for prolonged contact with the hip joint. The fossa and the atmospheric pressure work together to create a partial vacuum in the joint (Wingstrand et al., 1990).

1.1.1.2 The femur head and neck:

The femoral head is smooth and rounded. It forms two thirds of a sphere and is covered by hyaline cartilage. It is thick on the medial-central surface and thin on the periphery (Kempson et al., 1971). Small ligament connect the head of the femur with the floor of the acetabulum (ligamentum capitis).The capitis (teres) ligament (Figure

4, 5) originates from the peripheral edges of both sides of the acetabular notch, passes under and medially to the transverse acetabular ligament (which some of its fibers blend) and inserts into the pit, or fovea, on the head of the femur. This triangular ligament is both intra-capsular and extra synovial, due to the encapsulation of the synovial membrane, which isolates it from both the cavity and the synovial fluid. The round ligament is not involved in stabilizing the hip joint. Its major function is to be a conduit for the blood supply (via a small branch from the obturator artery) to the femoral head (Fuss and Bacher, 1991). This ligament is not present in approximately 10% of all individuals (Tan and Wong, 1990).

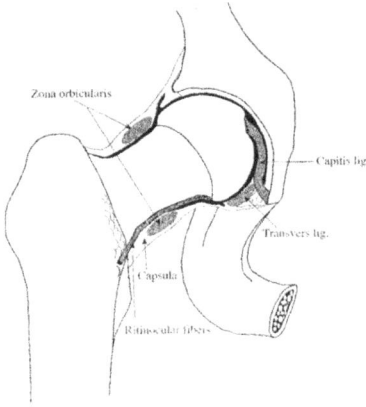

Figure 4: schematic drawing, showing the coronal section of the hip joint (author work).

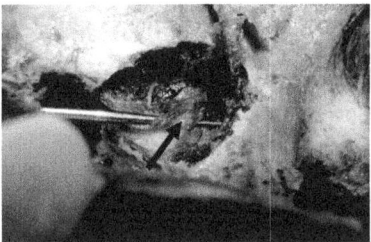

Figure 5: The round ligament of the head of the femur (arrow). Part of the acetabular bony walls were removed to expose the head from the inside (dissected by the author).

The neck of the femur is short (3-5 cm), cylindrical in shape (oval in cross-sectional) and attached to the shaft between the greater and lesser trochanter. The neck-to-shaft angle and angle of ante-version interact with the femoral shaft (Frankel, 1960). The neck-to-shaft angle (angle of inclination) occurs in the frontal plane and is measured between two lines; one axis passing through the femoral head and neck and the other through the shaft. The neck-shaft angle varies world-wide (ranging from $120°$ to $130°$) and is greater in males. This angle varies with age, beginning at $150°$ in young children and decreasing to $120°$ in the elderly. In adults, angulation over $135°$ is termed coxa valga and angulation below $120°$, coxa vara. An angle of torsion (also known as angle of anteversion) occurs in the transverse plane, and is measured between one axis passing through the distal femoral condyles and another axis passing through the femoral head and neck. This angle may vary from $10°$-$15°$. Anteversion refers to a pathological increase in the angle of torsion, and retroversion, to a decrease in the angle. As in the femoral neck-shaft angle, this angle also decreased with age; in the newborn it is approximately $40°$ and in the adult between $10°$ to $15°$. Femoral inclination and torsion angles are properties of the femur and exist independently of the hip joint. Therefore, abnormalities in the angulations of the femur can cause compensatory hip changes and can substantially alter hip joint stability, weight bearing biomechanics of the hip joint, and muscle biomechanics (Levangie and Norkin, 2001). Accordingly, such abnormalities should be considered in FHNLs studies.

Although the femoral head seems to fit perfectly into the acetabulum (congruent joint), there is substantially more articular surface on the head of the femur than on the acetabulum. Therefore, in a standing position, the articular surface of the femoral head remains exposed anteriorly and slightly superiorly. Because the inferior orientation of the acetabular does not align perfectly with the angle of inclination of the femur, the acetabulum does not fully cover the head superiorly. Furthermore, the anterior torsion of the femoral head is poorly matched to the anterior orientation of the acetabulum, exposing substantial amounts of the femoral head's anterior articular surface. When discrepancies between the angles of the femur and the acetabulum are considerable (as in cases of coxa valga), a large area of the femoral head's articular cartilage is exposed. This exposure causes a joint stability). Most importantly, maximum articular coverage of the femoral head is obtained when the femur is flexed, abducted, and laterally rotated, a position common in quadruped animals (Kapandji, 1987).

1.1.1.3 The hip joint capsule:

The hip joint capsule is the strongest and thickest capsule in the human body, supplying substantial stability to the joint (Figure 6). The thick sleeve is attached firmly around the rim of the acetabulum, in some parts to the labrum and to the edge of the obturator foramen.

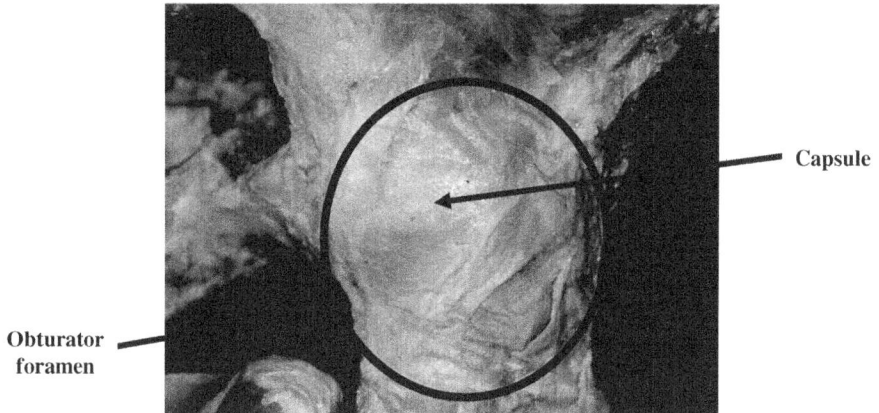

Figure 6: The hip joint capsule (dissected by author).

The capsule surrounds the neck of the femur, attaches to the trochanter line in the front and to the base of the neck above and behind. Some of the fibers reflect upwards along the neck as longitudinal bands (retinacula) and contain blood vessels that supply the head and neck of the femur (Figure 7a). The fibrous capsule, consisting of both circular and longitudinal fibers, is much thicker in its upper region, where the greatest amount of resistance is required (Figure7b).

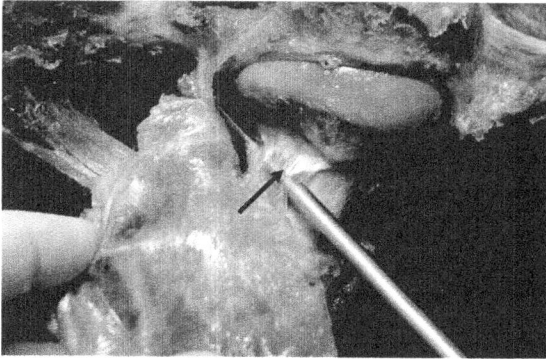

Figure 7a: The hip joint capsule retinacula (arrow) containing blood vessels that supply the head and the neck of the femur (dissected by author).

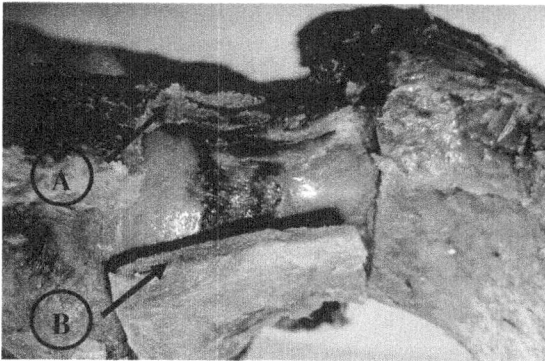

Figure 7b: The hip joint capsule: the thickness of the hip joint capsule is much greater in the upper superior part (arrows a, b) (dissected by author).

The circular fibers (zona orbicularis) (Figure 8) are the deepest and form a collar or ring (sling) around the neck of the femur. John et al. (2002) has suggested replacing the term "zona orbicularis" with "femoral arcuate ligament". This ligament is located in the deep capsular layer, on the posterior aspect of the hip. The arcuate ligament begins at the greater trochanter, proceeds to the ischiofemoral ligament, around the posterior circumference of the femoral neck, and inserts into the lesser trochanter.

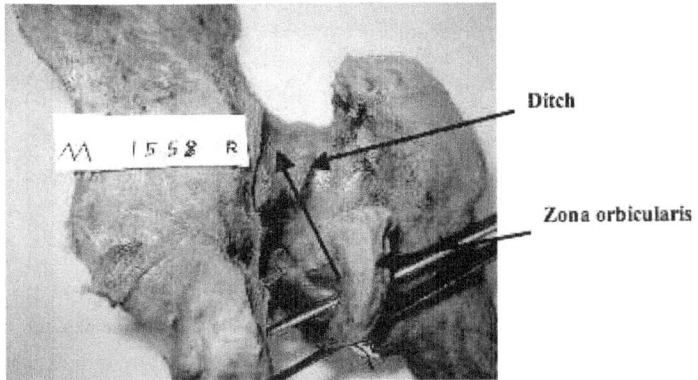

Figure 8: The zona obicularis separated from the hip joint capsule (arrows) (dissected by author).

In contrast to the zona orbicularis, the femoral arcurate ligament does not run continuously around the circumference of the capsule, but rather extends only halfway around the posterior aspect of the femoral neck (John et al., 2002). Its main function is to supply tension to the capsule .The more superficial layer consists of longitudinally oriented fibers and is much thicker than the zona orbicularis. Its thickest part is in the antero-medial part, where the fibers blend with the pubofemoral and ischiofemoral ligaments. The iliofemoral ligament further reinforces the capsule anteriorly. The major weakness of the capsule is located in its anterior region, between the iliofemoral and pubofemoral ligaments, where no ligaments or capsule fibers are present. The tendon of the iliopsoas muscle lies on top of the bursa. All the ligaments, but most particularly, the iliofemoral ligament, contribute to the stabilization and protection of the hip joint (Figure 9).

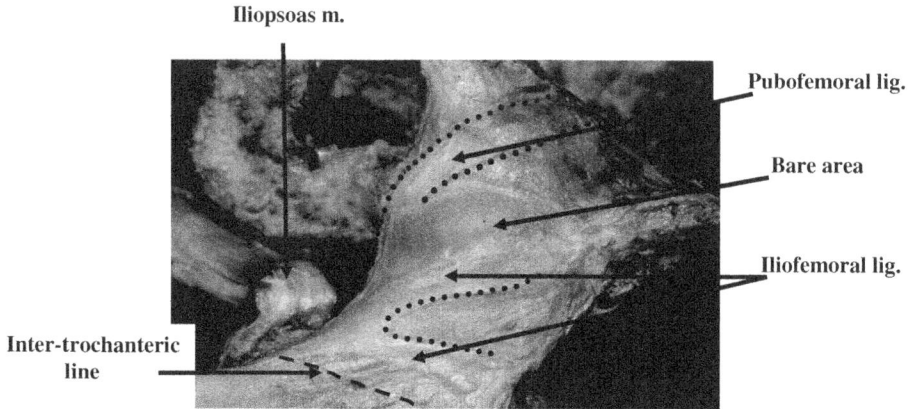

Figure 9: The capsule bare area, located between the iliofemoral and the pubofemoral ligaments, is the major weakness area of the hip joint. The tendon of the iliopsoas muscle crosses this area. A bursa is situated between the tendon and the capsule (author work).

The ligament, also called the Y-ligament of Bigelow, is triangular in shape and quite strong (Figure 10). Its upper part attaches superiorly to the anterior inferior iliac spine (AIIS) and to the body of the ilium between the AIIS and the acetabular rim. Distally, it divides into two bands: the superior band along the upper part of the intertrochanter line and the inferior band running downward and laterally along the lower part of the intertrochanteric line. The superior band of the iliofemoral ligament is the strongest and thickest of the hip joint ligaments. The capsule is thinner between the two bands of the iliofemoral and pubofemoral ligament (Figure 9). In some instances, there is no division, and the ligament stretches to become a flat triangular band, attached to the entire length of the intertrochanteric line.

The pubofemoral ligament (Figure 10) is attached to the body of the pubic bone near the acetabulum, and to the adjacent superior pubic ramus, which passes anteriorly to the head and the neck, merging with the capsule and the medial band of the illiofemoral ligament. The pubofemoral ligament assists in preventing hyperextension, as well as controlling excessive abduction of the thigh (Gray, 1985).

31

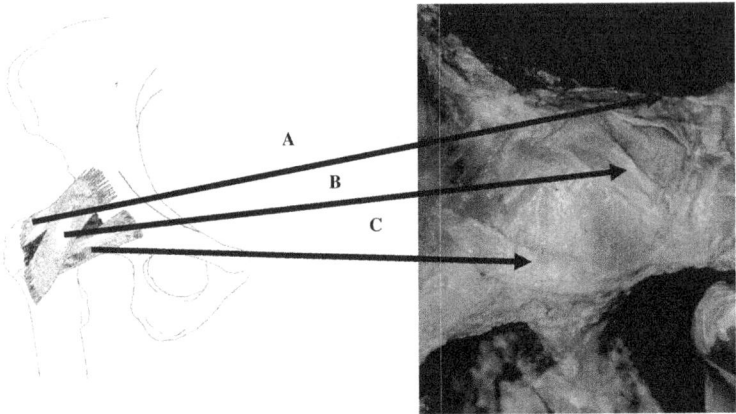

Figure 10: The Y-ligament (iliofemoral a&b) and pubofemoral (c) ligament. Note the differences between the classical anatomical description (left) and the actual position of the ligaments (author work).

The transverse acetabular ligament:

The transverse acetabular ligament (Figure 4) is a part of the acetabular labrum. It has no cartilage along its fibers, and runs along the periphery of the acetabulum on each side of the acetabular notch. Subsequently, it crosses the notch, and converts it into the foramen through which the nutrient vessels enter the joint. The two bands of the round ligament attach to the transverse acetabular ligaments. In a cross-sectional view, the ligament is triangular in shape. Externally it is in contact with the capsule, while internally it inclines inward, narrowing the acetabulum and embracing the cartilaginous surface of the head of the femur.

The ischiofemoral:

The ischiofemoral ligament (Figure 11) is triangular in shape and originates from the posterior aspect of the acetabular and the ischial bone. Its lower fibers blend with the circular fibers of the capsule (zona orbicularis) and insert into the femoral neck, just medial to the greater trochanter (some fibers are also inserted into the trochanteric fossa). Its upper fibers blend with the iliofemoral ligament. As with the other capsular ligaments, the ischiofemoral ligament tenses during extension of the femur, thereby restricting internal rotation and adduction when the hip is flexed.

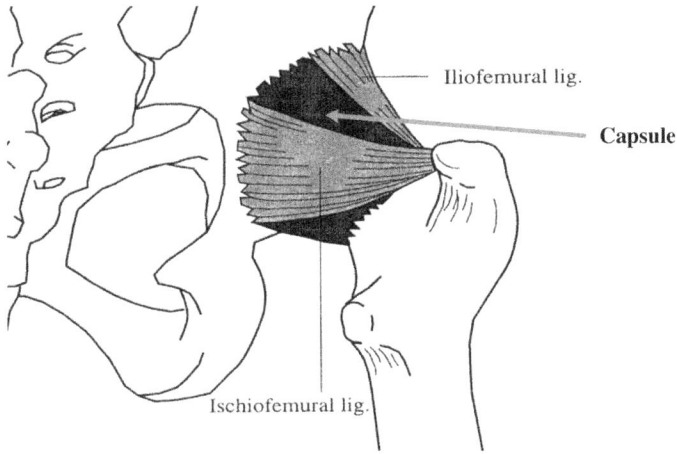

Figure 11: Posterior view of the hip joint. Note the location of the ischiofemoral ligament and its relation to the capsule (author work).

The synovial membrane

The synovial membrane begins at the border of the cartilaginous surface of the head of the femur. It extends over the portion of the neck contained within the joint capsule, both surfaces of the labrum, and the mass of fat in the depression of the acetabular fossa, and exposes the ligament of the head of the femur (round lig.). Occasionally, it is in contact with the subtendinous iliac bursa, lying deep to the tendon of the psoas major. When this occurs, there is anterior contact with the pubofemoral ligament and the more medial band of the iliofemoral ligament.

1.1.2 Major bony landmarks associated with the hip joint

The greater trochanter projects superiorly from the junction of the neck and the shaft of the femur. It consists of four facets (anterior, lateral, posterior and superoposterior) and serves as an attachment site for four muscles: the gluteus medius m, gluteus minimus m, piriformis m, and abturator internus m. The lesser trochanter projects from the posteromedial surface of the femur, distal to the neck, where the common tendon of the psoas major and iliacus m (iliopsoas m.) connects with the lesser trochanter.

The gluteal tuberosity is a roughened area located on the posterior surface of the femur at the superior end of the lateral lip of the linea aspera. Sometimes, the tuberosity becomes two osseous ridges. It is also the insertion area for the gluteus maximus m.

The trochanteric fossa is a depression located on the medial side of the greater trochanter, at the insertion site of the obturator internus m. and gemellus m.

The intertrochanteric line is an osseous ridge on the anterior surface of the femur, running obliquely and downward from the greater to the lesser trochanter, and attaching to the fibrous joint capsule.

The intertrochanteric crest is a heavy ridge on the posterior aspect of the femur, connecting the greater and lesser trochanters. The crest is the insertion site of the quadratus femoris.

1.1.3 The immediate structures around the hip joint

Anteriorly, the hip joint is in direct contact with the joint capsule, the bursae which underlie the iliacus, and the tendon of the psoas major. Anteromedially, some of the more lateral fibers of the pectineus muscle are in contact with the capsule. The femoral vesses and nerves are located more superficially, as are the rectus femoris m, sartorius m, and tensor fasciae latae m.

Superiorly, the reflected head of the rectus femoris muscle is adjacent to the more medial aspect of the capsule, while the gluteus minimus m. adheres closely to the lateral aspect. Inferiorly, the obturator externus, the lateral fibers of the pectineus, and the medial femoral circumflex artery are in close proximity to the joint.

Posteriorly, and near to the articular capsule are the obturator externus and internus, the gemelli, and the piriformis muscles. The quadratus femoris and gluteus maximus muscles are more superficial, as are the sciatic and posterior femoral cutaneous nerves. The gluteus maximus covers all of these structures.

1.1.4 Blood supply

Blood to the hip is supplied from three sources: (1) an extra capsular ring located at the base of the femoral neck (2) ascending cervical branches of the extracapsular ring on the surface of the femoral neck, and (3) the round ligament artery(branch of the obturator artery).

The extracapsular ring is supplied primarily by the medial femoral circumflex artery and ascending branch of the lateral femoral circumflex, both of which arise from the profunda femoris artery (Figure 12). The ascending cervical branches pierce the capsule and ascend along the osseus surface of the neck. The vessels terminate by penetrating the head at the junction of the articular cartilage. The femoral head receives its nourishment from blood vessels which travel primarily along a distal-proximal path, and which are prone to disruption in fracture, dislocation, and surgical approach (Gray, 1985).

1.1.5 Nerve supply

The femoral, obturator, and superior gluteal are the major nerves in the hip. Additional nerve branches connect to the quadratus femoris from the accessory obturator nerve and the lumbar sympathetic ganglia. The branches of the femoral nerve arise either directly from the nerve itself, or from its muscular branches that supply the iliofemoral ligament of the capsule, especially near its femoral insertion. The articular branch, originating from the obturator nerve, supplies the medial portion of the capsule, the pubofemoral area, and may reach the synovial tissue and ligament at the head of the femur. The nerve leading to the quadratus femoris supplies several fine branches to the ischiofemoral portion of the capsule near its femoral attachment. The superior gluteal nerve supplies fibers superolaterally to the capsule. Any sympathetic fibers from the lumbar ganglia that reach the hip joint follow the small articular vessels which penetrate the capsule (Gardner, 1948).

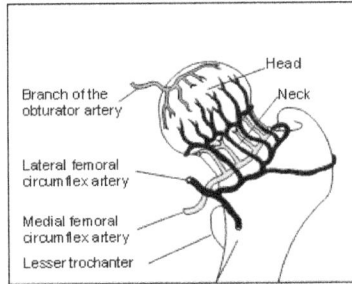

Figure 12: The femoral head neck blood supply (adapted from http://www.orthobethesda.com/education/understandingarthritis.aspx).

1.2 Hip joint anatomical anomalies related to femoral head-neck lesions (FHNL)

1.2.1 Coxa vara and coxa valga

Coxa vara (Figure 13) occurs when the angle of the femoral neck shaft decreases to less than 120°. Congenital coxa vara (CCV) is present at birth. CCV is assumed to result from either an embryonic limb bud abnormality or an intrauterine condition that causes significant proximal femoral varus. It is commonly associated with significant limb length discrepancy, segmental shortening of the femur, and other abnormalities of the bony femur. Associated diagnoses include proximal femoral focal deficiency, congenital short femur, and congenital bowed femur.

Coxa vara aids in improving hip joint stability. The apparent improvement in congruence occurs when the decreased angle between the neck and the shaft of the femur turns into the femoral head, deeper into the acetabulum, thus decreasing the amount of articular surface exposed superiorly and increasing coverage from the acetabulum. A varus femur, if not due to trauma, may also increase the length of the moment arm (MA) of the hip abductor muscle by increasing the distance between the femoral head and the greater trochanter. The increased MA decreases the amount of force that must be generated by the abductor muscles in single-limb support and reduces the joint reaction force. However, the coxa vara increases the bending moment along the femoral head and neck. This increase manifests in the increased density of trabeculae, laterally in the femur, due to the increase in tensile stresses

36

(Bombelli et al., 1984). The increased shear force along the femoral neck increases the predisposition toward femoral neck fracture (Singleton and Leveau, 1975; Radin, 1979).

Coxa vara may increase the likelihood of the femoral head sliding on to the cartilaginous epiphysis during adolescence. (Williams, 1995). Consequently, the superimposed weight compresses the head into the epiphyseal plate. In adolescence, growth of the bone results in a more oblique orientation of the epiphyseal plate. The epiphyseal obliquity makes the plate more vulnerable to shear forces at a time when it is already weakened by rapid growth (Lewinnek et al., 1980). Weight-bearing forces may slide the femoral head inferiorly, resulting in a slipped capital femoral epiphysis. As is true in hip fractures, the altered biomechanics and endangered blood supply require that normal alignment be restored before secondary degenerative changes can occur.

In coxa valga (Figure 13 b) the angle of inclination in the femur is greater than the normal adult angle of 125. The increased angle brings the vertical weight-bearing line closer to the shaft of the femur, diminishing the shear, or bending force. However, the decreased distance between the femoral head and the greater trochanter also decreases the length of the MA of the hip abductor muscle. The decreased muscular MA requires greater muscular force in order to maintain sufficient abduction torque. This subsequently counterbalances the gravitational adduction movement around the supporting hip joint during single-limb support. If the additional muscular force increases the total joint reaction force within the hip joint, the abductor muscle is unable to meet the increased demand and is thus functionally weakened. Although the abductors may be normal, the reduction in biomechanical effectiveness may result in compensation typical of primary abductor muscle weakness. Coxa valga also decreases the size of the femoral articular surface, in contact with the dome of the acetabulum. As the femoral head points more superiorly, the superior coverage from the acetabulum decreases. Consequently, coxa valga decreases the stability of the hip and predisposes the hip to dislocation (Kapandji, 1987; Singleton and Leveau, 1975; Radin 1979).

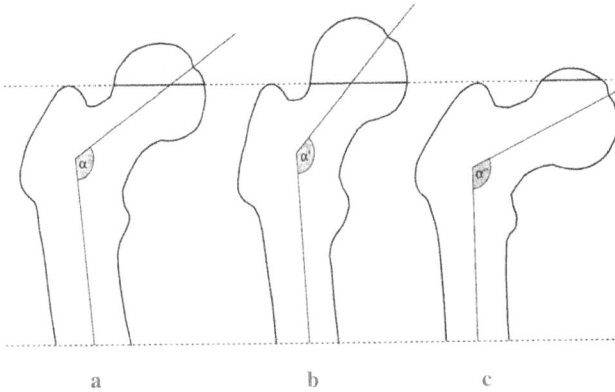

Figure 13: The neck-shaft angle (angle of inclination) occurs in the frontal plane between an axis through the femoral head and neck and the longitudinal axis of the femoral shaft: a- normal (average 125^0); b- coxa valga ($>130^0$); c- coxa vara ($<120^0$) (author work).

1.2.2 Anteversion and retroversion of the femur

Variation in the angle of torsion also affects hip biomechanics and function. Anteversion of the femoral head (Figure 14) reduces hip joint stability because the femoral articular surface is more exposed anteriorly. The line of hip abductors may drop more posteriorly to the joint, reducing the MA for abduction (Clark and Haynor, 1987). As is true for coxa valga, the resultant need for additional abductor muscle force may predispose the joint to arthrosis or may functionally weaken the joint, producing energy-consuming and wearing gait deviations. The effect of femoral anteversion may also be seen in the knee joint. When the femoral head is anteverted, pressure from the anterior capsuloligamentous structures and the anterior musculature may push the femoral head back into the acetabulum, causing the entire femur to rotate medially. Although the medial rotation of the femur improves the congruence in the acetabulum, the knee joint axis through the femoral condyles now turns medially, altering the plane of knee flexion/extention and resulting in a toe-in gait. The abnormal position of the knee joint axis and toed-in gait are commonly labeled medial femoral torsion. While medial femoral torsion and femoral anteversion both describe an exaggerated twist in the femur, femoral anteversion refers to an alteration

38

of the mechanics at the hip joint and medial femoral torsion, to an alteration at the knee joint. Femoral retroversion (Figure 14) is the opposite of anteversion.

Figure 14: Angle of torsion of the femur occurs in the transverse plane between an axis through the femoral head neck and an axis through the distal femoral condyles: I-normal torsion; II- anteversion, III-retroversion; intersecting line running parallel to the posterior femoral condyles and a line passing through the head and neck of the femur (adapted from Levangie and Norkin, 2001).

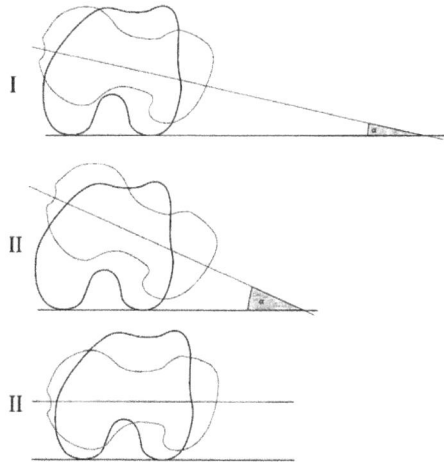

1.2.3 Anteversion and retroversion of the acetabulum

Retroversion of the acetabulum has been described as a posteriorly oriented acetabular opening, positioned in the sagittal plane. A retroverted acetabulum may occur as a result of posttraumatic dysplasia, or in association with bladder extrophy. A retroverted acetabulum has been identified as a cause of hip pain and a preosteoarthritic deformity. Acetabular retroversion generally acts as an obstacle to flexion and internal rotation of the hip by creating impingement of the anterosuperior aspect of the head and neck against the proximal-medial aspect of the acetabular rim. The manifestation of symptoms without a preceding trauma is usually activity-dependent and includes groin pain, which gradually increases over time. The morphology of acetabular retroversion is not uniform. The degree of overlap of the anterior aspect of the rim varies considerably. The more caudal portion of the acetabulum is more anteverted than the cephalic portion, as both the anterior and the posterior aspects of the acetabular rim run caudally in a spiral manner. Thus, measurements of the acetabular at the midpoint of the joint are unlikely to portray sufficiently acetabular version in the roof area, which is the crucial site for femoro-acetabular impingement and labral and cartilage rim lesions (Siebenrock et al., 2003). Identifying the normal acetabular anteversion is essential for proper implant positioning and preventing dislocation in total hip arthroplasty. The acetabulum is not a simple hemispheric shape. As a result, the acetabular anteversion angle would seem to be influenced by the point of measurement along a configuration that is possibly either curved or angular (Masaaki et al., 2001). The literature concerning the exact definition of the anteversion of the acetabulum is unclear. The anteversion is often defined as the angle between the acetabulum axis and the coronal plane of the body. The acetabulaum axis is perpendicular, and runs through the center of a line drawn between the end posterior margins. The average degree of anteversion of the acetabulum is approximately 17°, ranging from 11.5° to 28.5°. It is difficult to measure the degree of anteversion of the cup by roentgenographic examination. However, McLaren (1973) reported a mathematical method of determining the degree of anteversion whereby the relative position of the anterior and posterior halves of the circumferential wire in the cup is calculated. Superimposition of the two halves of the anterior suggests little or no anteversion. However, if an ellipse is formed, some degree of anteversion or retroversion can be seen.

1.2.4 Biomechanical notes

Even just standing on two legs loads the hip joint with a force equivalent to 30% of the body weight (Soderberg, 1986). When a person stands on one leg, the force imposed on the hip joint increase to approximately 2.5 to 3 times of the body weight (Saudek, 1985). In stairs climbing, hip joint force can reach levels of 3 times body weight and are on average 23% higher than walking (Bergmann el al., 2001). In walking, the force range from 2.5 to 7 times body weight and in running, the forces can be as high as 10 times body weight (Soderberg, 1986; Saudek, 1985). Yet, the hip joint can with stand 12 to 15 times body weight befor fracture in the osseous component occurs (Saudek, 1985).

The alignment of the femur relative to the acetabulum affects the loads applied to the hip joint. The joint reaction force on the head and neck of the femur during upright standing is more vertically aligned than the femoral neck, creating a bending moment on the head and neck of the femur (Maquet, 1999; Pauwels, 1976; Ruff, 1995). The bending moment produces tensile forces on the superior aspect of the femoral neck and compressive forces in the inferior aspect of the neck (Pauwels, 1976) (Figure 15). It is therefore why femoral necks with a wider superior inferior diameter can better handle the bending moment sustained during weight bearing. The trabecular arrays of bone found in the proximal femur are alignment to resist there compressive and tensile forces. When bone density decrease (osteoporosis) the risk of femoral neck fracture rises. Intrinsic alignment of the femur is on important element in the relationship between the femur and the acetabulum. The femoral head is directed forward the superior and the anterior aspect of the acetabulum. This is why measuring the neck-shaft angle (angle of inclination) is of significant important. The joint reaction force on the femur is more parallel to the femoral neck in coax valga. This alignment subjects the femoral neck to more compressive forces and less of a bending moment. The perpendicular distance between the hip joint center and the trochanter is decreased in coax valga, putting the hip abductors muscles at a disadvantage by reducing their moment arm. To overcome this disadvantage, these muscles must generate longer contractile forces to support the hip joint, resulting in increased joint reaction forces (Ruff, 1995). In addition, the joint reaction force in displaced laterally in the acetabulum and is applied over a smaller joint surface, leading to increase front stress. It is therefore why coxa valga are likely to increase the risk of degenerative hip joint disease. In coxa vara, in the other hand, the bending moment applied to the neck increase (Maquet, 1999). There the less in this deformity the trochanter is moved away from the joint center, lengthening the moment arm of the abductors, hence reduce the joint reaction force.

The problem with coxa vara is that it tends to increase the medial pull of the femur into the acetabulum, something that can contribute to the erosion of the acetabulum (Maquet, 1999).

Transverse plane alignment is also associated with proper function of the hip joint. Femoral anteversion for example assist in coping with forces acting mainly in the horizontal plane (Tayton, 2007). Excessive femoral anteversion, however, places the head of the femur further anteriorly in the acetabulum. This is being compensated by medial rotation of the hip resulting in in –toed posture. With time, however, many individuals with excessive femoral anteversion develop a secondary compensation in the foot laterally with respect to the knee. As a result, the in-toed standing posture disappears. Retroversion, on the other hand result in increased lateral rotation range of motion of the hip, the outcome of which is excessive out-toeing.

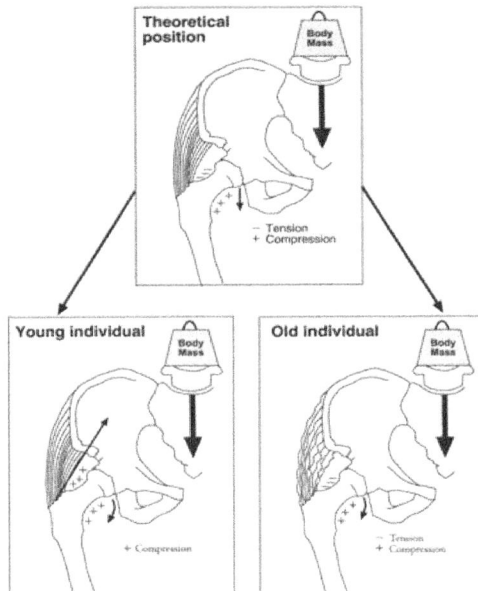

Figure 15: Tensile and compressive forces on the femoral neck from young to old individuals.

1.3. The acetabulum in humans and apes

There are considerable similarities in the anatomy of the hip joint in both humans and apes. The major differences relate to the joint design, i.e. acetabular orientation. In humans, the acetabular cavity faces obliquely forward, outward and downward, while in apes it faces horizontally outward; the anterior ligaments (iliofemoral, pubofemoral) and posterior ligament (ischiofemoral) in humans are twisted around the femoral neck in the same direction, while in apes the ligaments are weaker and run in a straight line between their two points of attachments (Aiello and Dean, 1990); there is large variation in acetabular depth among apes (Schultz, 1969), while humans manifest a much shallower acetabular than chimpanzees and gorillas, yet deeper than orangutans; the human acetabulum also has a differente ratio of the acetabular notch width to the acetabular diameter; the size of the acetabulum relative to body size is larger in humans than in apes.

1.4. The anthropological perspective of FHNL

There is a great ambiguity in the anthropological and anatomical literature in regard to the terminology associated with FHNLs. Historically, the most renowned FHN lesion is Allens' fossa, named after the anatomist who first illustrated the phenomenon in 1884 in his anatomical textbook, and named it the "Cervical fossa". This fossa was later named "anterior cervical imprint", or "bourrelet cotyloidien" of Poirier, a name rejected by Meyer (1934) on the ground that 'bourrelet' implies a prominence or a cushion and therefore cannot be used to designate a fossa. Meyer (1934) himself suggested to call the fossa "imprint of Bertaux" and not Allens' fossa, since Bertaux was the first to give a detail anatomical description of the phenomenon. The cervical (Allen) fossa is a depression located at the anterior superior margin of the femoral neck, close to the femoral head. The fossa varies in size and shape among individuals (Finnegan, 1978; Odgers, 1931), and may be expressed as "a mere depression to an area of removal of cortical bone one square centimeter in size, surrounded by slightly raised borders..." (Angel, 1964, p. 130). Poirier (1911) called this fossa "empreinte iliaque" (Meyer 1934). Walmsley (1915) suggested the name "capsular groove" and its lateral edge which is often clearly defined by a bony ridge-the "capsular ridge" (the "bourrelet osseux" of Poirier). Walmsley (1915) claimed that the anterior femoral neck can generally be divided into two areas: an outer smooth area and an inner (medial) rough area, separated by a bony ridge (the "capsular ridge"). This ridge starts to appear at the age of 18 years and is progressive

43

in development, "yet varies with the amount and strength of the capsular fibers" (p. 308). Odgers (1931) divided the "empriente" into three cateogories: depression; slight erosion; marked erosion (similar to the divisions given by Pearson and Bell in 1919). Meyer (1934) claimed that this categorization is meaningless as they in fact present the same process and therefore should be regarded as one type of facet – depressions or fossae (p.485). It is note worthy that Walmsley (1915) identified two additional imprints on the lower margin of the femoral head, namely the "pubic imprint" and the "ischial imprint" which he called "facet of rest" (p. 311) which were never followed in future literature.

Another type of FHNL previously described is known as"Poirier's facet". It is a small and smooth bulging of the femoral head articular surface toward the anterior part of the femoral neck (Finnegan, 1978). The phenomenon was first described by Henke (1863) and later by Poirier (1911). Often times there is confusion between the "Poirier facet" and "Poirier's empreiente (Odgers, 1931). The 'eminentia' phenomenon was first described by Cruvellhier, 1862; Henle, 1871 and later described by Sudeck (1899). Fick (1904) suggested that the cartilage extension corresponded to a marked "beetartige Erhabenheit" which he called the "Eminentia articularis colli femoris".

Odgers (1931) claimed that Fick (1904) wrongly says that Poirier had already named the "empreinte iliaque". According to Odgers, there is confusion between an elevated ridge of bone and a depression (or erosion), being called the same thing in different languages. Pearson (1916) puts Poirier's facet, the empriente and the eminentia in the same category and describes them as a consequence of a prolonged biological process. Pearson and Bell (1919) described Poirier's facet and the reaction area (fossa and plaque) as types of the same phenomenon: alpha- 'unbroken prolongation of the articular surface on to the anterior face of the neck", beta – divided into two groups: (a) excavation type located where the facet is usually found and (b) excavation located down on the anterior surface of the neck…sharply defined edges frequently undercut … on the floor the cancellous bone is frequently exposed, and (c) gamma –

a rough impression situated on the anterior face of the neck, the facet proper of Poirier.

Meyer (1924) suggested a modified classification for FHNLs, based on stage of development: (a) Eminentia articularis colli femoris - a prolongation of the articular surface covered by hyaline cartilage, (b) a transitional form - alpha type of Pearson and Bell, similar to Poirier facet, (c) raised area - cervical ridge, (d) irregular depression, (e) a shallow deep sulcus or oval depression, (f) a roughened area. In a later article, Meyer (1934) refutes Pearson and Bell (1919) hypothesis and claimed that their type beta does not correspond with Allens' fossa. Odgers (1931) claim that the "eminentia" which he defined as a raised ridge of bone, practically always presents with different degrees of distinctness in all bones, stretching from the head of the femur to the superior tubercle of the intertrochanteric line (p.357). According to Odgers, the "eminentia" is seen more frequently in males than in females, and is missing in the gorilla, chimpanzee and gibbon. The medial portion of this ridge may be covered to a varying degree with an extension of fibro-cartilage from the head of the femur and is seen much more frequently in males (Odgers, 1931, p. 357). Meyers (1934) wondered about this statement as the articular cartilage on the head of the femur is hyaline. Furthermore, Meyer (1934) claimed that the above description by Odgers (1931) is false as he confused between 'eminentia articularis colli femoris' (described by Fick and later by Sudeck) and the longitudinal superior bone prominence that runs along the entire femoral neck, from the intertrochanteric line to the femoral head (Meyer suggested to call this anatomical structure 'torus cervicalis'). Further, its absence or presence does not condition articular prolongation (Poirier facet) or depression (Allens' fossa), although it may help bring the neck and the acetabular lip together. Kostick (1963) claimed that if the cervical ridge is absent it is very likely that Poiriers' facet will be lacking too. He also noted that the presence of cartilage is often taken as prerequisite for Poiriers' facet although Poirier (1911) and other earlier researchers (e.g., Odger, 1931) did not claim so.

In 1964 JL Angel published an article entitled "The reaction area of the femoral neck" where he adopted a more generalized perception of the various lesions stating

45

that there is a sensitive area on the anterior surface of the femoral medial end of the bar, and that this reaction area may appear either as a fossa or as a plaque. Angel argued that the difference between plaque and poiriers' facet is that the later is always covered by hyaline cartilage, whereas the plaque is covered by parts of the hip joint capsule reflected up over the surface of the femoral neck (rarely some fibrocartilage may appear on the plaque). Although Angel claimed that distinction between the two can be carried out also on dried bones, he did not supply any criteria. With the development of the "Non-Metric" traits variation concept (Bery and Bery, 1967, 1971), the FHNLs were grouped under this title (Finnegan, 1978). Finnegan supplied an osteological definition for "Allen's fossa", "Poirier facet" and "Plaque". Nevertheless, he did not go into the pathophysiology of these non-metric traits, nor did he describe possible relationships between the three. Finnegan tried to shed light on the difference between Poirier facet and plaque: Poirier's facet is located at the same area where Allen's fossa is. The plaque formation is an extension of the articular surface of the femoral head toward the neck and has rounded margins (Finnegan, 1978).

In summary, anthropologists have defined four major femoral head and neck lesions (FHNLs): Allen's fossa, Poirier's Facet, plaque formation, and posterior cervical imprint. Allen's fossa is a local, usually rounded defect located at the anterior-superior margin of the femoral neck, close to the margin of the head. It can be large or small, and is usually expressed as a deep, oval depressed area, with sharp margins. Its floor can be smooth or eroded and trabeculae may sometimes be seen. Poirier's facet is an expansion or bulging of the articular surface of the head toward the upper anterior portion of the femoral neck. This upsurge bony plate is usually leaf-like in shape, with a narrowing neck connecting it to the head. It usually manifests well-defined margins. This facet is necessarily smooth, and is not to be confused with plaque formation (Poirier, 1911; Kostick, 1963; Finnegan, 1978). Plaque formation was described by Finnegan (1978). It is an overgrowth from the area of Poirier's facet towards the femoral neck, where it can cover Allen's fossa. Posterior cervical imprint was first described by Walmsley (1915) and later by Kostick (1963). It resembles Poirier's facet, but is located on the posterior aspect of the femoral neck.

As there is no sharp distinction between the various lesions and because the pathophysiology is uncertain, confusion exists in the literature. The terms for anterior cervical imprint, Allen's fossa, Berteaux imprint and Poirier facet are used interchangeably. Kostick, following previous suggestions made by Pearson and Bell (1919), suggested dividing these imprints into two types:

Type A: an ulcer-like excavation with floor and edges, that may, in some cases, manifest a clean, punched-out appearance, with sharp edges and a depressed floor.

Type B: a pleomorphic type, that presents as a discontinuity in the normal bony appearance of the neck, and is not definitely circumscribed. It may show a mouth-eaten or worn cancellous appearance, as though the cortical bone had been gradually erased (Kostick, 1963).

1.5. The medical perspective of FHNL

Although very common and of potentially high risk to the individual, FHNL has been largely ignored by the medical milieu. Very little information in the medical literature exists as to the frequency, etiology and pathophysiology of these lesions. This may be due to the fact that these phenomena are not usually recognized on radiographs. Although documented in skeletal material (Angel, 1964; Kostick, 1963), no systematic study has been carried out on these lesions and interpretations of them remain largely speculative.

In recent years, few studies presenting a possible relationship between FHNL and clinical signs and symptoms were published in the orthopedic literature.

1.5.1 Femoro-acetabular impingement (FAI)

Femoroacetabular impingement (FAI) is a condition of an increased friction between the acetabular rim and the femoral head neck junction, due to reduced anteversion at the anterolateral femoral head neck junction (Jager et al., 2004). Siebenrock et al. (2004) has suggested that abnormal extention of the articular surface of the femoral head (epiphyseal extension) correlates with decreased head-neck offset and a nonspherical appearance of the head. These, according to Siebenrock et al. (2004) expose the hips to risk of femoracetabular impingement (FAI) and subsequent osteoarthritis, especially in highly active individuals, who may repeatedly experience a forceful jamming of the nonspherical femoral head into the constrained acetabulum. The impingement can be seen intra-operatively after arthrotomy or can be demonstrated with an open arthro-magnetic resonance imaging technique, with the hip in maximum flexion and internal rotation (Siebenrock et al., 2003). In a dissection of the hip joint, Leunig et al. (2003) has shown rounded, ridge-like prominences of the anterolateral neck of the femur that extend from the head toward the greater trochanter.

On the basis of skeletal morphologic features, two distinct types of FAI have been identified. The first is caused by jamming an abnormally shaped femoral head, and the second is associated with acetabular misalignment, which increases acetabular contact between the acetabular rim and the femoral head-neck junction (Leunig et al., 2005; Siebenrock et al, 2004).

1.5.2 Fibrocystic changes of the femoral neck and synovial herniation pits

Recently, several studies used the reaction area (in the femoral neck) of Angel (1964) as a marker of pathological reactions in the femoral neck:

A. Synovial herniation pits: round, well-circumscribed lucent areas, located at the anterolateral cortex of the femoral neck. They may be related to the relationship between the hip joint capsule and the iliopsoas muscle, especially in athletes (Crabbe et al. 1992). The herniation pit, first described by Pitt et al. (1982) as histologic and radiologic entity, is found in asymptomatic patients and is considered a normal variant. This lesion has been related to a reaction area on the surface of the femoral neck, covered by dense collagenous tissues and fibro cartilage.

B. Fibrocystic changes of the femoral neck: is located at the anterosuperior femoral neck, surrounded by a narrow margin of sclerotic bone, and visible on conventional radiographs, computed tomographic scans (CT), magnetic resonance images (MRI), and even bone scan of the hip (Crabbe et al., 1992; Thomason et al., 1983). The origin of the fibrocystic change is related to common acquired change at the anterosuperior femoral neck. Hewitt et al. (2001) suggested that the Y ligament presses the anterosuperior aspect of the hip capsule when the hip is fully extended. Pitt et al. (1982) proposed that the synovial tissue herniates through a cortical bone defect of the femoral neck.

During the first three decades of the past century, Fick (1904), Poirier (1911), and Meyer (1924) offered different theories describing the origin of the herniation pits. Odgers (1931) was the first to suggest that the reaction area is in direct contact with the zona orbicularis when the capsule tightens in full extension (which may produce nonphysiologic stress on the bony bar). Leunig et al. (2005) indicated that there is a relationship between the herniation pit and the site of impingement.

C. Femoral osseous heads-neck deformity (FOHND): located on the anterolateral femoral head-neck junction. Stuhllberg et al. (1975) described this deformity as a "pistol-grip deformity." Its etiology is unclear, and it is thought to be a risk factor for osteoarthritis and femoroacetabular impingement. FOHND is associated with several disorders which are associated with an abnormal anatomical relation between the femoral head and neck, resulting in bump formation. The diagnosis of FOHND is based on standard radiographs of the proximal femur in two planes.

2. AIMS OF STUDY

The major purpose of the current study is to reveal the etiology and pathophysiology of the femoral head and neck lesions (FHNL).

The aims of the study are:

1) To redefine macroscopically the lesions of the femoral head and neck.

2) To reveal their association with demographic parameters (e.g., sex, age, ethnic origin).

3) To reveal their association with femoral architecture (e.g., neck-shaft angle, torsion).

4) To reveal their association with pelvis and acetabular architecture (e.g., anteversion, retroversion, volume (depth) etc.

5) To reveal their association with soft tissue hip joint structures (e.g., iliofemoral ligament, capsule thickness, zona orbicularis).

6) To present a model that will best describe the etiology of these lesions.

3. MATERIALS AND METHODS

3.1. The studied population

The hip joints of 524 adult (>20 years) human skeletons and 12 human cadavers were used in this study. The human skeletons were of modern populations from the Hamann-Todd Osteologic Collection (HTH), housed at the Laboratory of Physical Anthropology at the Cleveland Museum of Natural History, Ohio, USA. The HTH Collection includes 3100 well-documented human skeletons (known age at death, sex, race, cause of death, height and weight) of African-American and European-American males and females born between the years 1825 and 1910. Most individuals were of low socioeconomic status. The age, sex, and ethnic distribution of the sample are presented in Tables 3.1.1 and 3.1.2. The 12 human cadavers (6 males and 6 females) were obtained from the Department of Anatomy and Anthropology, Sackler Faculty of Medicine, Tel Aviv University. Most human cadavers were between 70 to 90 years of age.

Table 3.1.1 : The studied sample (HTH-collection) by age and ethnic origin (adults only)

| Age | Ethnic origin | | Combined |
	African American	European-American	African-American and European-American
20-39	94	84	178
40-59	107	105	212
60+	55	79	134
Total	256	268	524

Table 3.1.2 : The studied sample (HTH-collection) by gender and ethnic origin (adults only)

| Gender | Ethnic origin | | Combined |
	African-American	European-American	African-American and European-American
Males	145	177	322
Females	111	91	202
Total	256	268	524

3.2. Types and definitions of lesions studied:

In the present study, we decided to remove ourselves from previous terminology and use a simple yet highly reliable method for categorizing FHNLs that can be applied to dry bones. We set up criteria for describing each trait with additional supporting pictures.

1) The 'Ditch' type (Figure 16): Defined as a basin on the anterior aspect of the femoral neck close to the margin of the femoral head, with defined bony margins. The ditch type may be subdivided into three stages of development: a) 'slight'- a shallow fossa with undefined margins and a smooth intact bony floor; b) 'intermediate'- a concavity with well defined margins and a floor manifesting early erosive changes with preliminary trabecular exposure; c) 'developed' – a deep, cup-shaped fossa (trench-like) with well defined margins, a floor manifesting advanced erosive changes (cribriform), and exposed trabeculae.

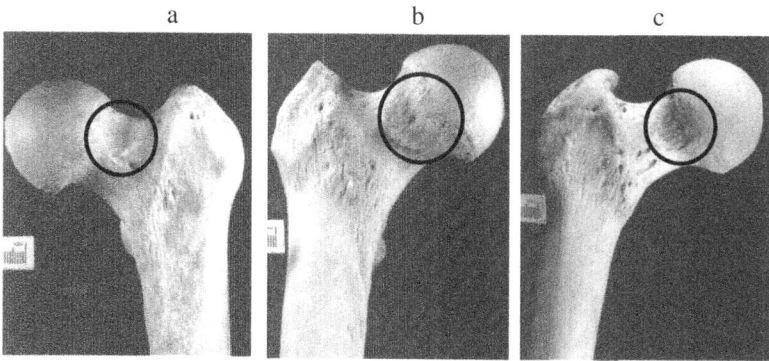

Figure 16: The "ditch" type lesion in the femoral neck: a- slight, b- intermediate and c- developed (circle) (author work).

2) <u>The 'Tongue' type</u> (Figure 17): Defined as an expansion from the articular surface of the femoral head to the upper anterior part of the neck. This slightly concave expansion is usually, although not necessarily, a leaf-like shape with a narrowed neck connecting to the head, usually with well-defined margins. The tongue type can also appear on the posterior aspect of the neck.

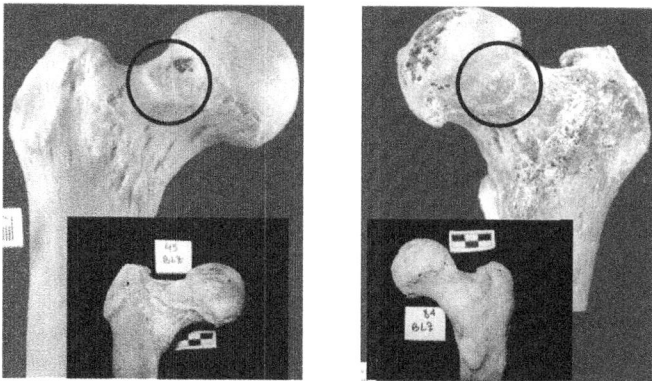

Figure 17: The "tongue" type in the femoral head and neck: a- the lesion on the anterior aspect, b- the lesion on the posterior aspect (circle) (author work).

3) The 'Indentate' type (Figure 18): Defined as a large, localized defect on the anterior-inferior part of the femoral head. Part of the head is carved out, damaging the spherical shape of the head. The defect is manifested as an inverted "U" shape, becoming wider and deeper inferiorly towards the neck. Its surface is usually smooth, although trabeculae may be exposed. In many cases, it appears together with the tongue type, creating a hook or S-like contour.

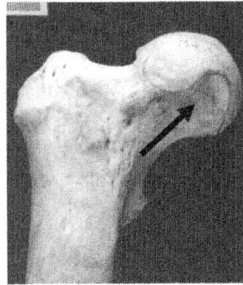

Figure 18: The indentate type in the femoral head and neck (arrows) (author work).

4) The 'Sunken' type (Figure 19): Defined as a local defect located at the lower anterior-inferior margin of the femoral head. This defect can be categorized as large or small, and usually appears as a deep, ovular depressed area with sharp margins. Its floor can be smooth or eroded, and trabeculae may occasionally be seen.

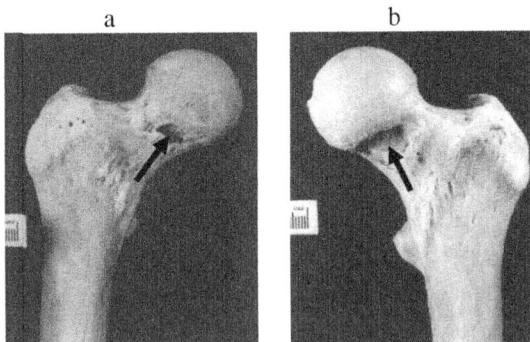

Figure 19: The "sunken" type of the femoral neck: a- small defect and b- large defect (arrows) (author work).

5) <u>The 'Groove' type</u> (Figure 20): Elongated deep groove along the anterior aspect of the femoral head, close to its margin. The groove is dug into the articular surface of the femoral head and possesses a clear margin, but no thickened osseous rim. The groove can reach considerable size in length and depth. The femoral head-neck junction is preserved.

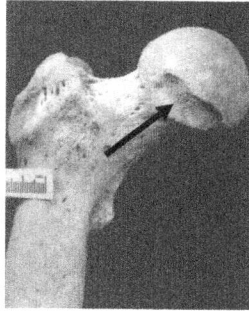

Figure 20: The 'Groove' type at the femoral head (arrow) (author work).

6) <u>The 'Pit' type</u> (Figure 21): Appears mainly on the anterior lower aspect of the femoral head, close to its margin. It is usually oval in shape, small in size (1.5X1.5 cm), clearly demarcated and relatively deep. Trabeculae may be exposed.

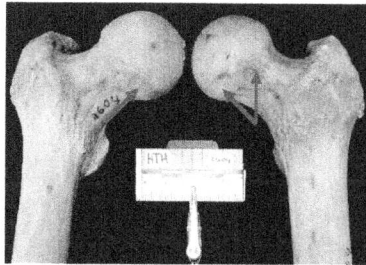

Figure 21: The 'Pit' type of the femoral head: small pit formation (arrows) (author work).

3.3. Femoral measurements (skeletal material)

Angular measurements were taken with a simple protractor. For linear measurements of large bones (femur, pelvis), we used a simple osteometric board, constructed of 1mm graph paper and a free moving ruler.

3.3.1 Linear measurements

For linear measurements such as femoral neck diameter and femoral head diameter, a sliding caliper was used.

Five anthropometric linear measurements of the femur were taken: anatomical length, trochanteric height, head diameter, neck diameter, neck length minimum, and neck length maximum (Figure 22).

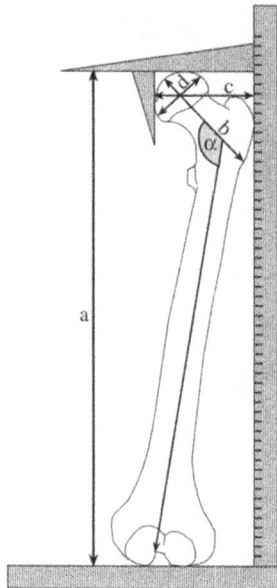

Figure 22: Measurements taken on the femur: a- anatomical length; b- maximum length of femoral neck; c- minimum length of femoral neck; d- head diameter; α- neck-shaft angle (author work).

3.3.2. Angular measurements

One angular anthropometric was taken: neck-shaft angle (coxa vara/valga) (Figure 22).

3.3.3 Femoral head torsion (Figure 23): The femur is placed on its posterior aspect on the base of the measuring device, and the moveable bar (pointer) is placed on the highest point of the femoral head. The distance is recorded (Peleg et al. 2007).

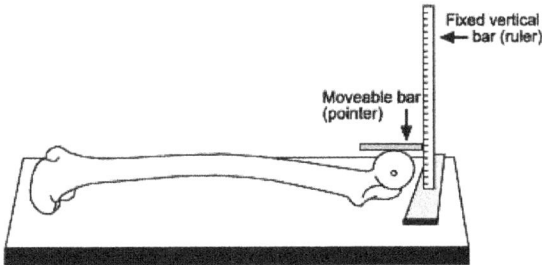

Figure 23: Measurement of femoral head torsion adapted from: Peleg et al., 2007

3.3.4. Femoral shaft bowing angle (new measurement) (Figure 24): The femur is placed on its posterior border on the base of the measuring device, and the moveable bar (pointer) is placed on the proximal femur (point e), distal femur (point a), highest (point b), and lowest point (point d) at the mid-femoral shaft.

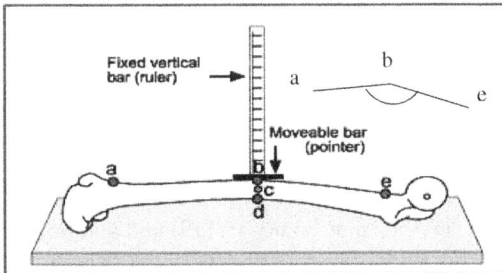

Figure 24: Measurement of femoral shaft bowing: a- distal shaft, b- midpoint of the shaft of the femur (top), c- midpoint between b and d, d- midpoint of the shaft of the femur (bottom), e- proximal shaft (author work).

3.4. Pelvic measurements

Anatomical reconstruction of the pelvis was accomplished with the help of strong rubber bands (see appendix 17).

3.4.1. Pelvic width (Figure 25): The pelvis was positioned on the osteometric board base, resting on its anterior superior iliac spines (ASIS) and anterior superior corners of the symphysis pubis. The iliac crests were placed against the fixed horizontal bar (ruler). The most lateral border of the pelvis was placed against the fixed vertical bar. A moveable bar was placed against the most lateral border of the other side. The distance was read from the osteometric board ruler.

Fixed horizontal bar (ruler)

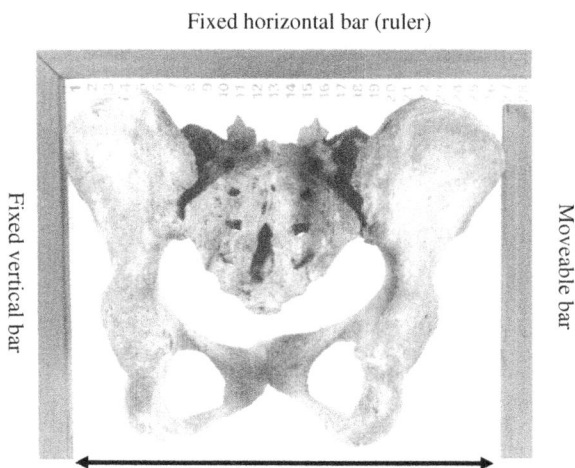

Figure 25: Measurement of pelvic width using osteometric board (adapted from: Peleg et al., 2007).

3.4.2. Pelvic height (Figure 26): The pelvis was positioned on the osteometric bord base, resting on its anterior superior iliac spines (ASIS) and anterior superior corners of the symphysis pubis. The ischial tuberosities were placed against a fixed horizontal bar. One lateral border was placed against a fixed vertical bar (ruler). A moveable bar

58

was placed against the uppermost borders of the pelvis. The distance was read from the osteometric board ruler.

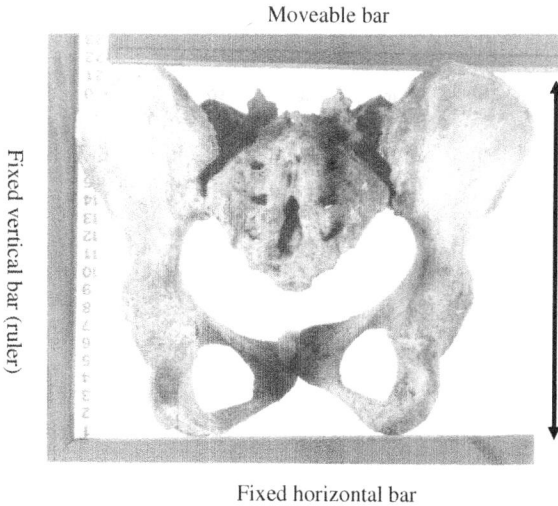

Figure 26: Measurement of pelvic height using osteometrec board (Adapted from: Peleg et al., 2007).

3.4.3. Pelvic inner measurement: Several measurements of the pelvis and the acetabulum were carried out using a Microscribe 3D (Figure 27) apparatus (Immersion Co. San Jose, CA). The Microscribe 3D was designed to create three-dimensional data, using the X, Y, and Z coordinates for anatomical landmarks. Microscribes are commonly used for anthropometric measurements and their validity has been proven in many studies (e.g., Peleg et al., 2007; Masharawi et al., 2008). To minimize positional distortion and ensure proper position, the pelvis was placed on a flat horizontal surface (ASIS and pubis in contact with the surface), ensuring proper coronal alignment, while the ischial tuberosities were in contact with a vertical plate, thus ensuring horizontal alignment. The symphysis pubis and midsacral points positioned on a marked line running perpendicular to the vertical plate ensuring proper sagittal orientation (Figure 27). A special metal device was used to properly stabilize the pelvis, avoiding minor movements during measurement. After calibrating the X, Y, Z coordinates of a fixed origin point to 0,0,0 respectively, the telescopic stylus of the apparatus was positioned at two defined anatomical landmarks (a, b) on the sacrum and one point (c) on the midsagittal line (Figure 28). A foot pedal (connected to the Microscribe) was pressed to enter the data into a previously designed Excel program. The computer then calculated anterior superior iliac spine width =ASISW (Figure 29a), sciatic notch width ScNW (Figure29a), Bi-acetabular rim distance= BARD (Figure 29a), bi-acetabular depth distance= BADD, posterior-superior iliac spine width= PSISW (Figure 29b), posterior inferior iliac spine width= PIISW (Figure 29b), ischial spine width =ISW (Figure 29b) acetabular inclination angle (Figure 30), acetabular version angle (Figure 31) and sacral inclination angle (Figure 32). The resolution and accuracy of the Microscribe as defined by the manufacturer were 0.13 mm and 0.43mm (mean values), respectively.

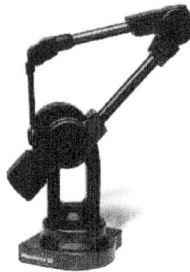

Figure 27: Microscribe 3D apparatus used in our study (Immersion Co. San Jose, CA).

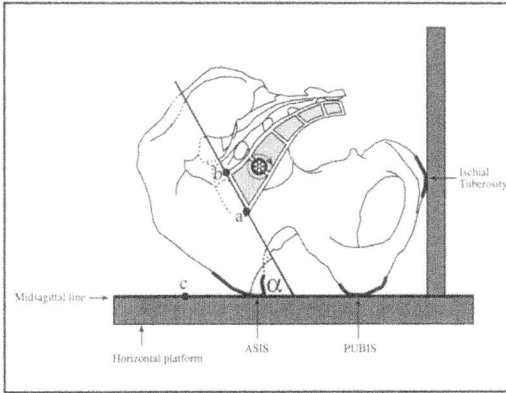

Figure 28: Points (a,b,c) recorded for sacral inclination measurement.

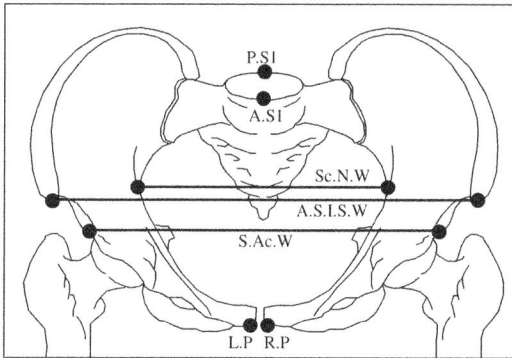

Figure 29a: Various measurements on the anterior aspect of the pelvis, carried out via the microscribe. Black dots mark the anatomical landmarks where the telescopic stylus was positioned (author work).

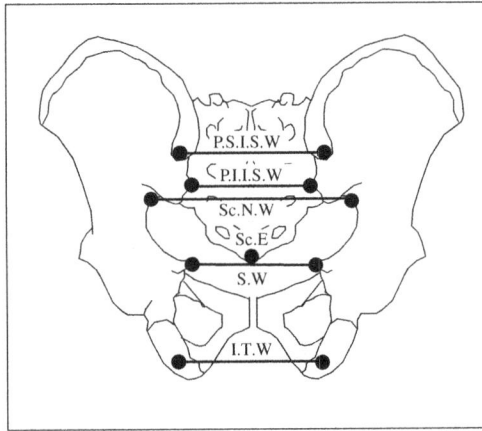

Figure 29b: Various measurements on the posterior aspect of the pelvis, carried out via the microscribe. Black dots mark the anatomical landmarks where the telescopic stylus was positioned (author work).

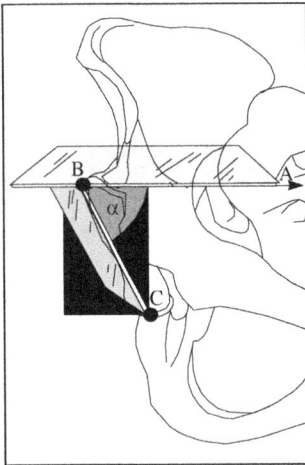

Figure 30: Measurement of acetabular inclination angle using the microscribe (author work).

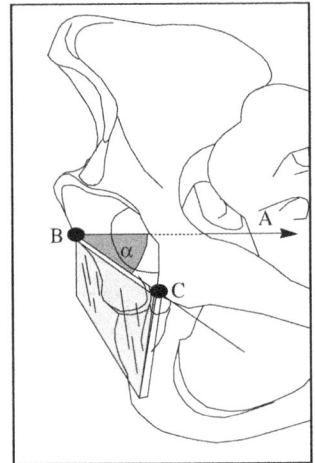

Figure 31: Measurement of acetabular version angle using the microscribe (author work).

3.4.4.Sacral inclination (Figure 32): Sacral inclination is defined as the angle created between one line running parallel to the superior surface of the sacrum (Figure 31, line a-b-e) and a second line running between the anterior superior iliac spine (ASIS) and the anterior-superior edge of the symphysis pubis (Figure 31, line c-d-e, angleα) (Peleg et al., 2007).

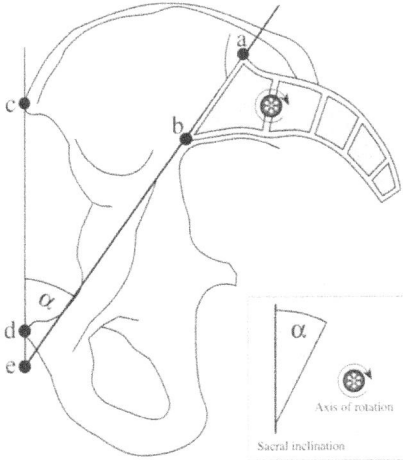

Figure 32: Definition of sacral inclination angle (adapted from: Peleg et al., 2007).

A special measuring device was designed in order to measure sacral inclination (Figure 32). A long bar was attached to a base at a 90° angle. A protractor was attached by a movable clamp to maintain a permanent 90° angle to the bar. A non-flexible bar was attached at the axis of the protractor (Peleg et al., 2007).

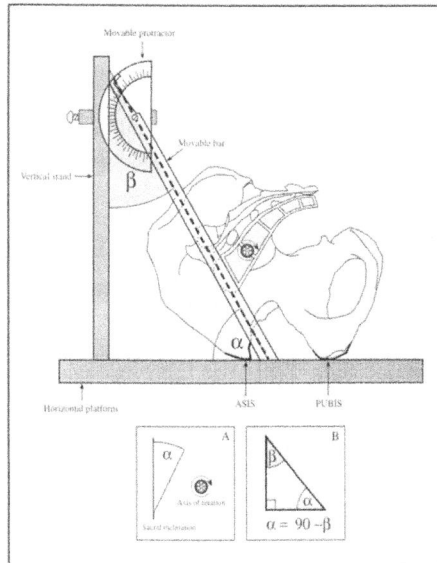

Figure 33: Measurement of sacral inclination using the specially designed device (adapted from: Peleg et al., 2007)

3.4.5. Pelvic incidence angle: Four anatomical points were used to calculate this angle: two on the superior surface of the first sacral vertebra (a, b, and Figure 33) and two at the centers of the acetabuli (AL, AR, and Figure 34). The two centers of the acetabuli were measured in two different ways: a- as the deepest (most medial) acetabular concavity (Ac. Depth.) and, b- as an average of the points on the line crossing the acetabulum from the most superior to the most inferior point and a similar point on the line running from the most posterior to the most anterior point (Figure 35). The femoral head axis in the original method was replaced by the acetabular axis (Whitesides and Horton, 2005; Mays 2006; Peleg et al., 2007).

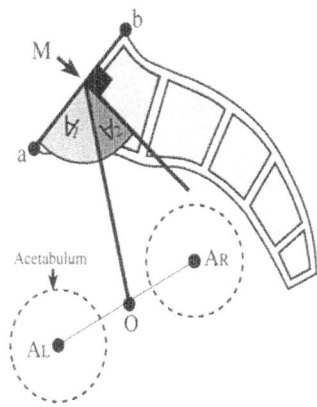

Figure 34: Measurement of pelvic incidence using the microscribe (adapted from: Peleg et al., 2007).

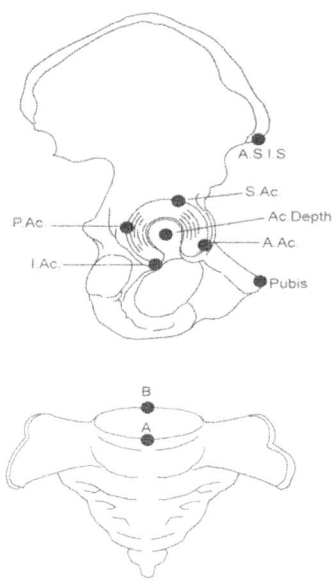

Figure 35: Points recorded by the microscribe for locating the center of the acetabulum.

3.5. Soft tissue analysis:

On each cadaver, a pelvicfemoral unit (PFU) was prepared as follows: first, we made a parasagittal section using an electric saw to cut through the sacroiliac joint, separating the inominates in each side. Then, we made a transverse section of the femur at its proximal mid-third. To reach the capsule and the ligament of the hip joint (Figure 36), we used scalpel and chirurgic tweezers to clean the surrounded tissue (skin, fat, muscles and vessels).Then; we made a transverse section on the level of the acetabular labrum and a sagittal section through the bare area to look for the femoral head-neck lesions (Figure 37).

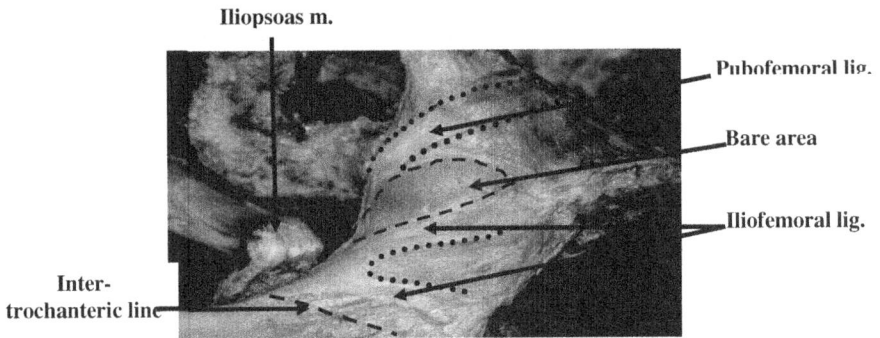

Figure 36: The hip joint capsule and ligaments (arrows) (author work).

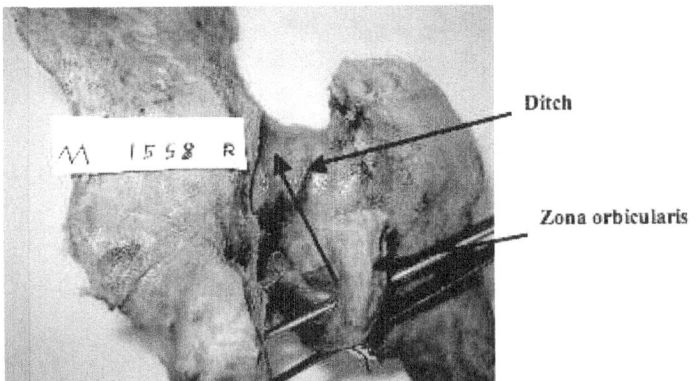

Figure 37: An open hip joint FHN lesion can be observed (arrows) (author work).

3.6. Statistical analysis:

Multivariate analysis, Pearson correlation, and chi-square tests were applied to demonstrate the association of the dependent variables (various FHNLs) with the independent variables (main size and shape of the femur, pelvis and acetabulum), as defined in the "Aims of the Study" chapter. The reconstruction of linear measures from the 3-D data obtained with the digitizer was accomplished with standard formulae (based on analytic geometry). All formulae were validated by Peleg et al. (2007) (Figure 38).

Calculating acetabular version and inclination angles (Figure 13, 14).

$$distance = \sqrt{(x_1 - x_2)^2 + (y_1 - y_2)^2 + (z_1 - z_2)^2}$$

$$angle\,\alpha = ar\cos\left[\frac{(x_1 - x_2)\,(x_2 - x_3) + (y_1 - y_2)(y_2 - y_3) + (z_1 - z_2)(z_2 - z_3)}{D_{b-a} * D_{b-c}}\right.$$

$$D_{b-c} = distance \rightarrow b \leftrightarrow c$$
$$D_{b-a} = distance \rightarrow b \leftrightarrow a$$

Calculating sacral inclination. Due to the occasional unevenness of the superior surface of the first sacral vertebra (i.e., "dome-shaped" sacrum) (Legaye et al., 1998), two different calculations were applied (Peleg et al., 2007), namely:

1. $\alpha_1 = degree[a\cos(Ay-By)]/D$

2. $\alpha_2 = degree[a\sin(Az-Bz)]/D$

When $D = \sqrt{((B_x - A_x)^2 + (B_y - A_y)^2 + (B_z - A_z)^2)}$

Figure 38: Calculations of acetabular version angle, acetabular inclination and sacral inclination angle.

Stages of calculating pelvic incidence. The calculation procedure is carried out in four successive stages (Peleg et al., 2007).

First stage: Measuring the location of points a and b on the sacrum (as in SI) and of the center of the acetabulum (A_R and A_L) using the 3-D digitizer.

$AR=(X_{AR}, Y_{AR}, Z_{AR})$

$AL=(X_{AL}, Y_{AL}, Z_{AL})$

$a=(X_a, Y_a, Z_a)$

$b=(X_b, Y_b, Z_b)$

Second stage: Calculating the central position of the sacral surface (M) and of the central point on the acetabular axis (O).

$$O = (x_O, y_O, z_O) = \left(\frac{X_{AR} + X_{AL}}{2}, \frac{Y_{AR} + Y_{AL}}{2}, \frac{Z_{AR} + Z_{AL}}{2} \right)$$

$$M = (x_M, y_M, z_M) = \left(\frac{X_a + X_b}{2}, \frac{Y_a + Y_b}{2}, \frac{Z_a + Z_b}{2} \right)$$

Third stage: Calculating the angle created at the intersection between the line a-b and O-M:

$$\cos \theta = \cos \alpha_1 \cos \alpha_2 + \cos \beta_1 \cos \beta_2 + \cos \gamma_1 \cos \gamma_2$$

When: $\cos\alpha$, $\cos\beta$ and $\cos\gamma$ are the cosinus of the vector's direction.

Calculating the cosinus of the vectors OM and ab directions:

OM length:

$$p(\underline{OM}) = \sqrt{(x_M - x_O)^2 + (y_M - y_O)^2 + (z_M - z_O)^2}$$

The direction's cosinus are:

$$\cos \alpha_{OM} = \frac{(x_M - x_O)}{p(\underline{OM})}, \quad \cos \beta_{OM} = \frac{(y_M - y_O)}{p(\underline{OM})}, \quad \cos \gamma_{OM} = \frac{(z_M - z_O)}{p(\underline{OM})}$$

<u>ab</u> Length:

$$p(\underline{ab}) = \sqrt{(x_a - x_b)^2 + (y_a - y_b)^2 + (z_a - z_b)^2}$$

The direction's cosinus are:

$$\cos \alpha_{ab} = \frac{(x_a - x_b)}{p(\underline{ab})}, \quad \cos \beta_{ab} = \frac{(y_a - y_b)}{p(\underline{ab})}, \quad \cos \gamma_{ab} = \frac{(z_a - z_b)}{p(\underline{ab})}$$

Then:

$$\forall 2 = \cos^{-1}(\cos \alpha_{OM} \cos \alpha_{ab} + \cos \beta_{OM} \cos \beta_{ab} + \cos \gamma_{OM} \cos \gamma_{ab})$$

Stage 4: Then the A1 is: $\forall 1 = 90 - \forall 2$

4. RESULTS

4.1: Demography of femoral head-neck lesions (FHNL).

4.1.1. General prevalence of FHNL (Table 4.1.1, Figure 39).

Among the 524 individual examined in the study, only 27.1% showed no lesions on the femoral head-neck. 32.3% exhibited tongue, 29.4% ditch, 3.1% indentation, 1.5% sunken, 4% combination of tongue and ditch, 1.5% groove and 1.1% pit.

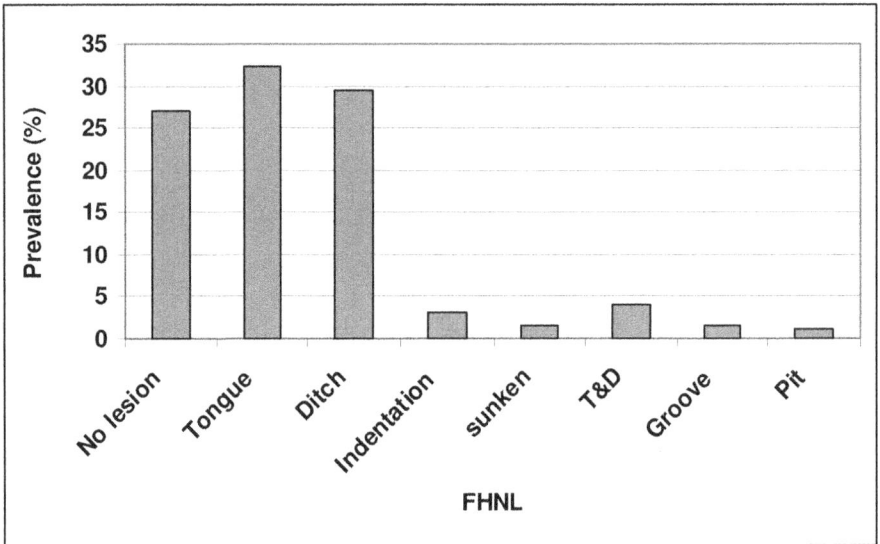

Figure 39: Prevalence of FHNL, general population.

4.1.2. Prevalence of FHNL in males and females (Table 4.1.1, Figure 40).

The distribution of FHNL differs significantly (P=0.030) between males and females. In general, there are more lesions in males compared to females (78% of all males manifested FHNL vs. 65% of females). Among males, the tongue type lesion was more prevalent than the ditch type (37% vs. 27%). However, in females, the opposite was observed (24% had tongue type lesions and 34% had ditch type). The combination of tongue and ditch type lesions was observed mainly in males (6.2%). In females this combination of lesions was relatively rare (0.5%).

Table 4.1.1: Prevalence of FHNL by sex.

Lesions	Sex				Sex Combined	
	Males		Females			
	N	%	N	%	N	%
No lesion	71	22	71	35.1	142	27.1
Tongue	120	37.3	49	24.3	169	32.2
Ditch	86	26.7	68	33.7	154	29.3
Indentation	15	4.7	1	0.5	16	3.1
Sunken	2	0.6	6	3	8	1.5
Tongue and ditch	20	6.2	1	0.5	21	4
Groove	4	1.2	4	2	8	1.5
Pit	4	1.2	2	1	6	1.1
Total	322	100	202	100	524	100

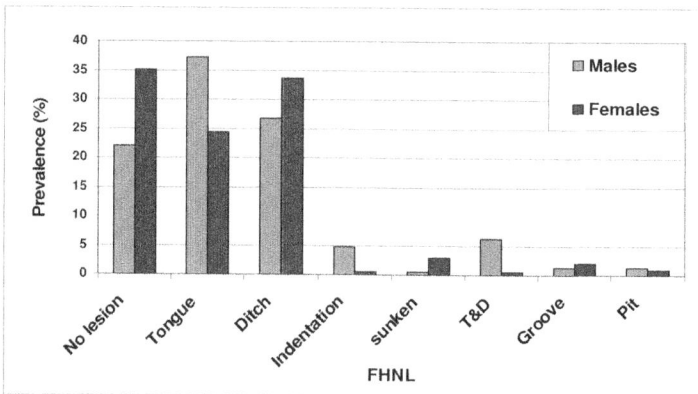

Figure 40: Prevalence of FHNL by sex.

71

4.1.3. Prevalence of FHNL in African-American (AfAm) vs. European-American (EuAm) (Table 4.1.2, Figure 41).

The distribution of FHNL by ethnic origin did not vary significantly (P=0.063).

Among AfAm, the ditch type was more common than the tongue type: 31.6% vs. 26.2%. Among EuAm the opposite situation was found, the tongue type was more prevalent than the ditch type 38.1% vs. 27.2%. When compared, the tongue type was more prevalent among EuAm (38.1%) than AfAm (26.2%).

Table 4.1.2: Prevalence of FHNL by ethnic origin, sex combined.

Lesions	Ethnic groups				Ethnic Combined	
	African-American		European-American			
	N	%	N	%	N	%
No lesion	72	28.1	70	26.1	142	27.1
Tongue	67	26.2	102	38.1	169	32.2
Ditch	81	31.6	73	27.2	154	29.3
Indentation	9	3.5	7	2.6	16	3
Sunken	5	2	3	1.1	8	1.5
Tongue and ditch	13	5.1	8	3	21	4
Groove	6	2.3	2	0.7	8	1.5
Pit	3	1.2	3	1.1	6	1.1
Total	256	100	268	100	524	100

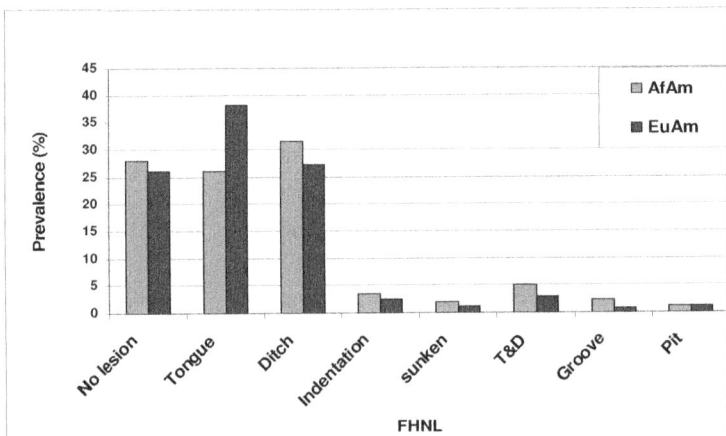

Figure 41: Prevalence of FHNL by ethnic origin.

4.1.4. Prevalence of FHNL by ethnic origin, males only (Table 4.1.3, Figure 42).

The distribution of FHNL in the male population did not vary significantly between the two ethnic groups (P=0.079).

For each ethnic group separately, AfAm males manifested a high prevalence of tongue type lesions (32%) followed by the ditch type (26%). EuAm males manifested similar trend: a high prevalence of the tongue type (41%) and a lesser prevalence of the ditch type (28%). When the two groups were compared, the tongue type was more prevalent among EuAm males (41%) compared to AfAm males (32%).

Table 4.1.3: Prevalence of FHNL in AfAm and EuAm, males only.

Lesions	Ethnic				Ethnic Combined	
	African-American Males		European-American Males			
	N	%	N	%	N	%
No lesion	35	24.1	36	20.3	71	22.0
Tongue	47	32.4	73	41.2	120	37.2
Ditch	37	25.5	49	27.7	86	26.7
Indentation	8	5.5	7	4	15	4.6
Sunken	1	0.7	1	0.6	2	0.6
Tongue and ditch	12	8.3	8	4.5	20	6.2
Groove	3	2.1	1	0.6	4	1.2
Pit	2	1.4	2	1.1	4	1.2
Total	145	100	177	100	322	100

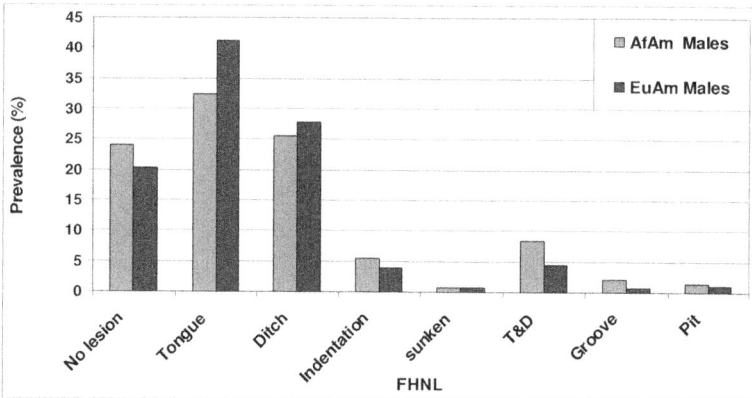

Figure 42: Prevalence of FHNL in AfAm vs. EuAm, males only.

73

4.1.5. Prevalence of FHNL by ethnic origin and sex, females only (Table 4.1.4, Figure 43).

The distribution of FHNL among females in the two ethnic groups did not vary significantly (P=0.079).

In AfAm females, the ditch type was much more common (40%) than in EuAm females (26%). The tongue type was more prevalent in EuAm females (31.9%), compared to AfAm females (18%). In AfAm females, the ditch type was significantly more prevalent than the tongue type (40% vs. 18%), while among EuAm females the tongue type was more prevalent than the ditch type (32% vs. 26%).

Table 4.1.4: Prevalence of FHNL in AfAm and EuAm, females only.

Lesions	Ethnic groups				Ethnic Combined	
	African-American Females		European-American Females			
	N	%	N	%	N	%
No lesion	37	33.3	34	37.4	71	35.1
Tongue	20	18	29	31.9	49	24.2
Ditch	44	39.6	24	26.4	68	33.6
Indentation	1	0.9	-	-	1	0.4
Sunken	4	3.6	2	2.2	6	2.9
Tongue and ditch	1	0.9	-	-	1	0.4
Groove	3	2.7	1	1.1	4	1.9
Pit	1	0.9	1	1.1	2	0.9
Total	111	100	91	100	202	100

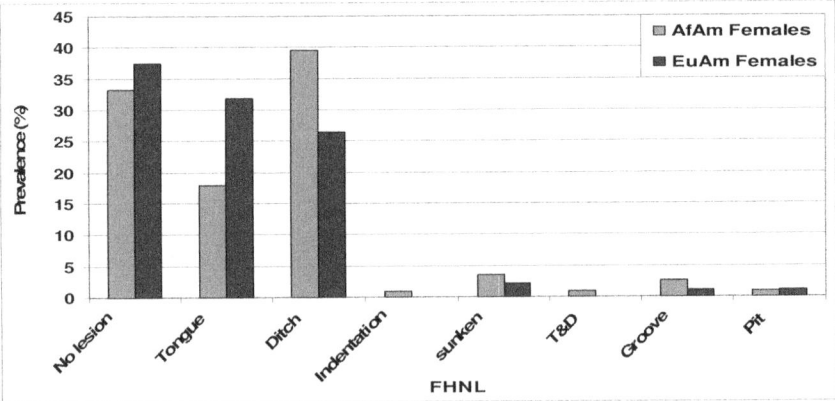

Figure 43: Prevalence of FHNL in AfAm and EuAm, females only.

4.1.6. Prevalence of FHNL in AfAm males and females (Figure 44).

The distributions of FHNL in AfAm males and females were similar (P=0.208).

When comparing AfAm males to AfAm females, the tongue type was more commonly found in AfAm males (32%) than in females (18%). The ditch type was more common in AfAm females (40% vs. 26%). AfAm males manifested a high prevalence of tongue type lesion (32%) followed by the ditch type (26%). By contrast, AfAm females were more likely to present the ditch type (40%), while only 18% presented with the tongue type.

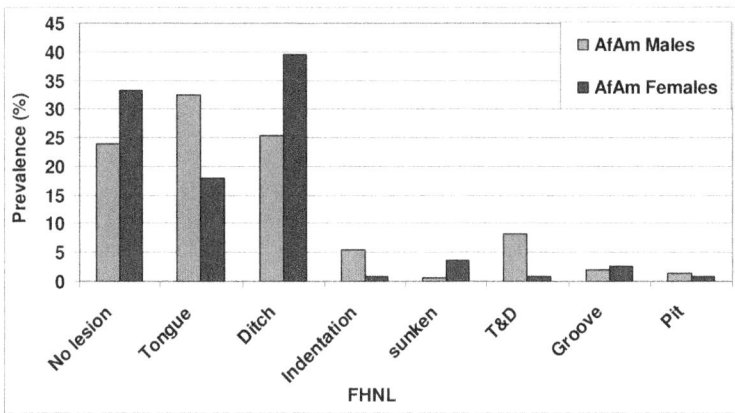

Figure 44: Prevalence of FHNL in AfAm males and females.

4.1.7. Prevalence of FHNL in EuAm males and females (Figure 45).

The distributions of FHNL in the EuAm males and females differed significantly (P=0.028).

When comparing EuAm males to EuAm females, the tongue type was more prevalent among the males (41% vs. 32%).

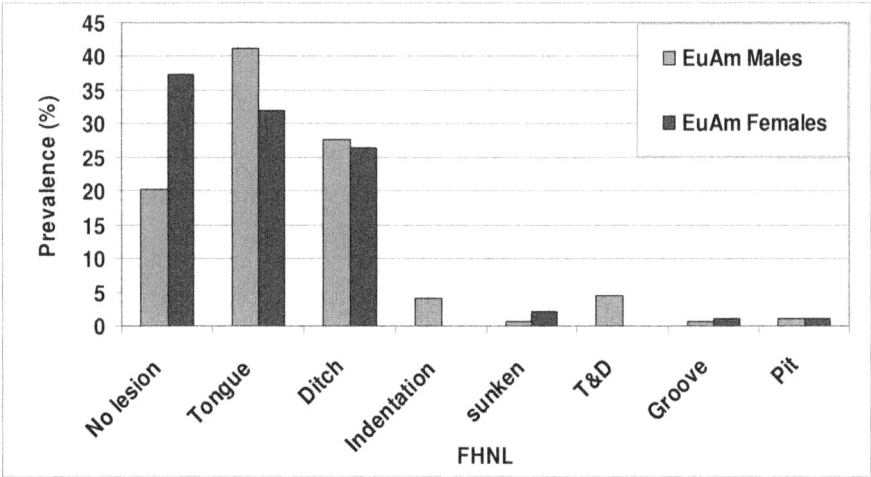

Figure 45: Prevalence of FHNL in EuAm males and females.

4.1.8. Prevalence of FHNL by age (Table 4.1.5, Figure 46)

The prevalence of the tongue type increased with age: 24.2% in the 20-39 age cohort, 34.4% in the 40-59 age cohort and 39.6% in the 60+ age group. The ditch type, on the other hand decreased in prevalence: 34.8% in the 20-39 age cohort, 29.7% in the 40-59 age cohort and 21.6% in the 60+ age cohort. The association of indentate, sunken, groove and pit types with age could not be examined due to the small sample size.

Table 4.1.5: Prevalence of FHNL by age.

Lesions	Age groups						Age combined	
	20-39		40-59		60+			
	N	%	N	%	N	%	N	%
No lesion	54	30.3	52	24.5	36	26.9	142	27
Tongue	43	24.2	73	34.4	53	39.6	169	32.2
Ditch	62	34.8	63	29.7	29	21.6	154	29.3
Indentation	2	1.1	10	4.7	4	3	16	3
Sunken	4	2.2	3	1.4	1	0.7	8	1.5
Tongue and Ditch	5	2.8	10	4.7	6	4.5	21	4
Groove	4	2.2	1	0.5	3	2.2	8	1.5
Pit	4	2.2	-	-	2	1.5	6	1.1
Total	178	100	212	100	134	100	524	100

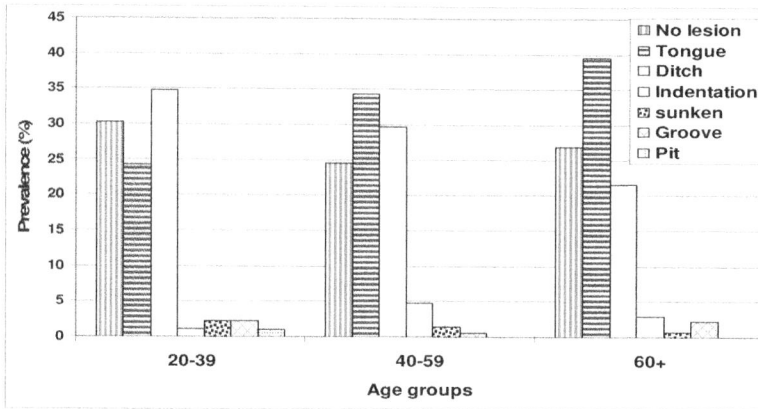

Figure 46: Prevalence of FHNL by age

4.1.9. Prevalence of FHNL by age, males only (Table 4.1.6, Figure 47).

When only males were considered, the tongue type prevalence increased with age, while the ditch type decreased. The prevalence of the indentate, sunken, and groove types did not vary with age.

Table 4.1.6: Prevalence of FHNL by age, males only.

Lesions	Males						Combined	
	Age groups							
	20-39		40-59		60+			
	N	%	N	%	N	%	N	%
No lesion	25	26.9	28	19.7	18	20.7	71	22
Tongue	27	29	52	36.6	41	47.1	120	37.2
Ditch	29	31.2	42	29.6	15	17.2	86	26.7
Indentation	2	2.2	9	6.3	4	4.6	15	4.6
Sunken	-	-	1	0.7	1	1.1	2	0.6
Tongue and Ditch	5	5.4	9	6.3	6	6.9	20	6.2
Groove	2	2.2	1	0.7	1	1.1	4	1.2
Pit	3	3.2	-	-	1	1.1	4	1.2
Total	93	100	142	100	87	100	322	100

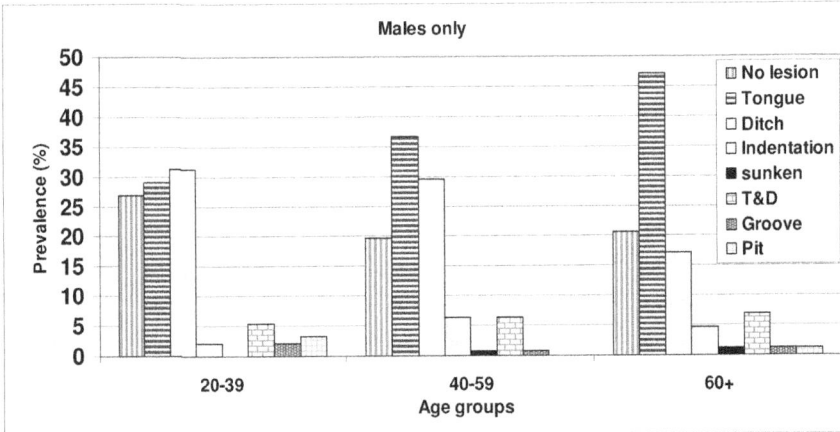

Figure 47: Prevalence of FHNL by age, males only.

4.1.10. Prevalence of FHNL by age, females only (Table 4.1.7, Figure 48).

Among females, the prevalence of the tongue type increased in the middle age group (30%) and decreased slightly in the elderly group (26%), while the prevalence of the ditch type decreased from the young group (38.8%) to the middle group (30%) and the old group (29%). The prevalence of the other types did not vary with age.

Table 4.1.7: Prevalence of FHNL by age, females only.

Lesions	Females						Age Combined	
	Age group							
	20-39		40-59		60+			
	N	%	N	%	N	%	N	%
No lesion	29	34.1	24	34.3	18	38.3	71	35.1
Tongue	16	18.8	21	30	12	25.5	49	24.2
Ditch	33	38.8	21	30	14	29.8	68	33.6
Indentation	-	-	1	1.4	-	-	1	0.4
Sunken	4	4.7	2	2.9	-	-	6	2.9
Tongue and Ditch	-	-	1	1.4	-	-	1	0.4
Groove	2	2.4	-	-	2	4.3	4	1.9
Pit	1	1.2	-	-	1	2.1	2	0.9
Total	85	100	70	100	47	100	202	100

78

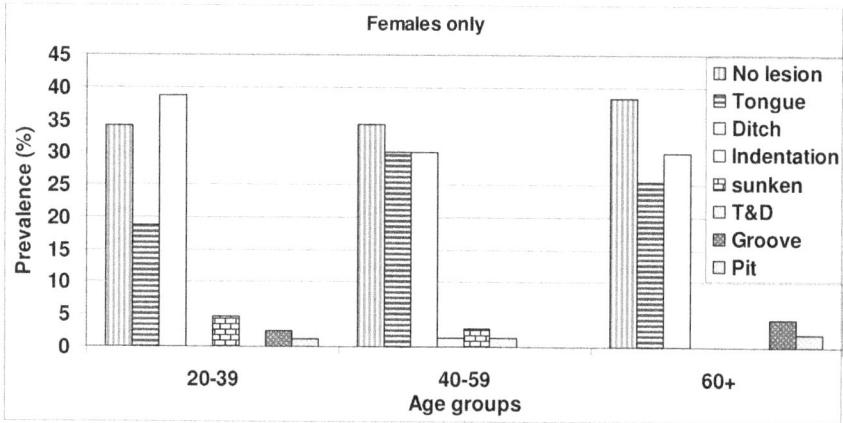

Figure 48: Prevalence of FHNL by age, females only.

4.1.11. Prevalence of FHNL by age, AfAm only (Table 4.1.8, Figure 49).

In AfAm, the tongue type prevalence increased from the young group (17%) to the middle age group (33%), and then decreased in the elderly age group (29%). The ditch type prevalence decreased from the young age group (37.2%) to the middle age group (30%), and continued to decrease in the old age group (26%). Other lesions did not vary with age.

Table 4.1.8: Prevalence of FHNL by age, AfAm only.

Ethnic	African-American						Combined	
	Age group							
Lesions	20-39		40-59		60+			
	N	%	N	%	N	%	N	%
No lesion	31	33	26	24.3	15	27.3	72	28.1
Tongue	16	17	35	32.7	16	29.1	67	26.1
Ditch	35	37.2	32	29.9	14	25.5	81	31.6
Indentation	-	-	6	5.6	3	5.5	9	3.5
Sunken	2	2.1	2	1.9	1	1.8	5	1.9
Tongue and Ditch	4	4.3	6	5.6	3	5.5	13	5
Groove	3	3.2	-	-	3	5.5	6	2.3
Pit	3	3.2	-	-	-	-	3	1.1
Total	94	100	107	100	55	100	256	100

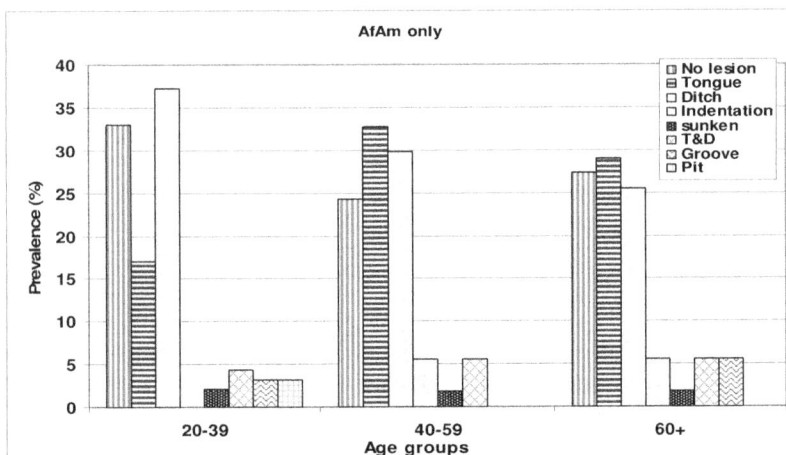

Figure 49: Prevalence of FHNL by age, AfAm only.

4.1.12. Prevalence of femoral head-neck lesions by age, EuAm only (Table 4.1.9, Figure 50).

In EuAm the prevalence of the tongue type increased with age, while that of the ditch type decreased with age. Other lesions did not vary with age.

Table 4.1.9: Prevalence of femoral head-neck lesions by age, EuAm only.

Ethnic	European-American						Combined	
	Age group							
Lesions	20-39		40-59		60+			
	N	%	N	%	N	%	N	%
No lesion	23	27.4	26	24.8	21	26.6	70	26.1
Tongue	27	32.1	38	36.2	37	46.8	102	38
Ditch	27	32.1	31	29.5	15	19	73	27.2
Indentation	2	2.4	4	3.8	1	1.3	7	2.6
Sunken	2	2.4	1	1	-	-	3	1.1
Tongue and Ditch	1	1.2	4	3.8	3	3.8	8	2.9
Groove	1	1.2	1	1	-	-	2	0.7
Pit	1	1.2	-	-	2	2.5	3	1.1
Total	84	100	105	100	79	100	268	100

80

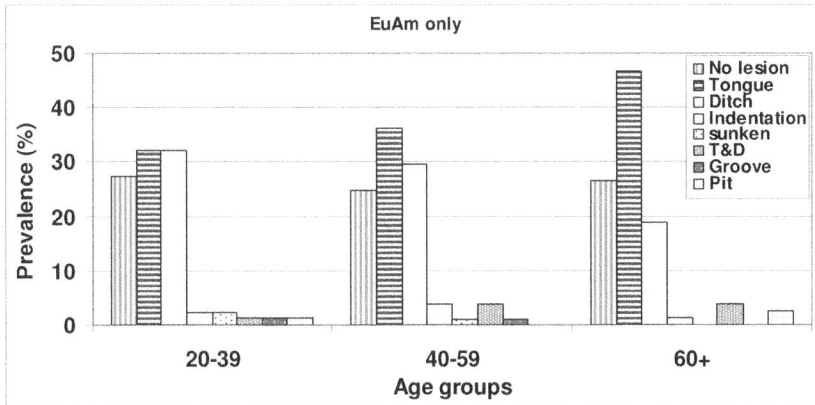

Figure 50: Prevalence of FHNL by age, EuAm only.

4.1.13. Prevalence of FHNL by age in AfAm males and females (Table 4.1.10).

When comparing AfAm males to females by age, AfAm males showed an increase in prevalence of tongue type with age, while AfAm females showed a sharp increase in the middle age group, followed by a sharp decrease in the older age group. The prevalence of the ditch type increased in the middle age and decreased in the older age group, while in females, the ditch type decreased significantly in the middle age group, yet increased significantly in the older age group.

Table 4.1.10: Prevalence of FHNL by age in AfAm males and females.

Age group	Lesions	African -American				Combined	
		Males		Females			
		N	%	N	%	N	%
	No lesion	14	33.3	17	32.7	31	32.9
	Tongue	9	21.4	7	13.5	16	17
	Ditch	11	26.2	24	46.2	35	37.2
	Indentation	-	-	-	-	-	-
20-39	Sunken	-	-	2	3.8	2	2.1
	Tongue and Ditch	4	9.5	-	-	4	4.2
	Groove	2	4.8	1	1.9	3	3.1
	Pit	2	4.8	1	1.9	3	3.1
	Total	42	100	52	100	94	100
	No lesion	13	19.7	13	31.7	26	24.2
	Tongue	23	34.8	12	29.3	35	32.7
	Ditch	20	30.3	12	29.3	32	29.5
	Indentation	5	7.6	1	2.4	6	5.6
40-59	Sunken	-	-	2	4.9	2	1.8
	Tongue and Ditch	5	7.6	1	2.4	6	5.6
	Groove	-	-	-	-	-	-
	Pit	-	-	-	-	-	-
	Total	66	100	41	100	107	100
	No lesion	8	21.6	7	38.9	15	27.2
	Tongue	15	40.5	1	5.6	16	29
	Ditch	6	16.2	8	44.4	14	25.4
	Indentation	3	8.1	-	-	3	5.4
60+	Sunken	1	2.7	-	-	1	1.8
	Tongue and Ditch	3	8.1	-	-	3	5.4
	Groove	1	2.7	2	11.1	3	5.4
	Pit	-	-	-	-	-	-
	Total	37	100	18	100	55	100

4.1.14. Prevalence of FHNL by age in EuAm males and females (Table 4.1.11).

When comparing EuAm males to females by age, EuAm males showed a similar prevalence of the tongue type in the young and middle age groups (35.3%, 34.8%), followed by a significant increase in the old age group (52%). EuAm females showed an increase in the tongue type within the increasing age groups (27.3%, 29.3%, and 37.9%). The prevalence of the ditch type in males decreased with age (35.3%, 30.3%, and 18%), while in females it increased in the middle age group (29.3%), and then decreased in the old age group (20.7%).

Table 4.1.11: FHNL frequencies by age in EuAm males and females.

Age group	Lesions	European -American				Combined	
		Males		Females			
		N	%	N	%	N	%
20-39	No lesion	11	21.6	12	36.4	23	27.3
	Tongue	18	35.3	9	27.3	27	32.1
	Ditch	18	35.3	9	27.3	27	32.1
	Indentation	2	3.9	-	-	2	2.3
	Sunken	-	-	2	6.1	2	2.3
	Tongue and Ditch	1	2	-	-	1	1.1
	Groove	-	-	1	3	1	1.1
	Pit	1	2	-	-	1	1.1
	Total	**51**	**100**	**33**	**100**	**84**	**100**
40-59	No lesion	15	19.7	11	31.7	26	24.2
	Tongue	29	34.8	9	29.3	35	32.7
	Ditch	22	30.3	9	29.3	32	29.9
	Indentation	5	7.6	-	2.4	6	5.6
	Sunken	-	-	-	4.9	2	1.8
	Tongue and Ditch	5	7.6	-	2.4	6	5.6
	Groove	-	-	-	-	-	-
	Pit	-	-	-	-	-	-
	Total	**76**	**100**	**29**	**100**	**105**	**100**
60+	No lesion	10	20	11	37.9	21	26.5
	Tongue	26	52	11	37.9	37	46.8
	Ditch	9	18	6	20.7	15	18.9
	Indentation	1	2	-	-	1	1.2
	Sunken	-	-	-	-	-	-
	Tongue and Ditch	3	6	-	-	3	3.7
	Groove	-	-	-	-	-	-
	Pit	1	2	1	3.4	2	2.5
	Total	**50**	**100**	**29**	**100**	**79**	**100**

4.1.15. General frequencies of FHNL by side (Figure 51).

The tongue and the ditch lesions appeared on both the right and left femur with similar frequencies, 81.1% and 82.5% respectively. In 7.1% of the individuals with the tongue type lesion, the lesion appeared also in the posterior aspects of the femoral proximal epiphysis.

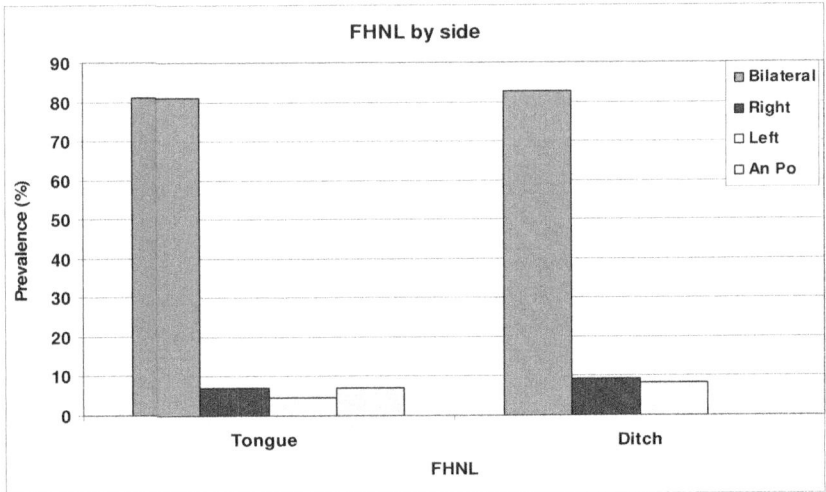

Figure 51: Prevalence of FHNL by side.

4.1.16. Major demographical findings:

1). There are more FHNL in males than females.

2). In males the tongue type lesion is the most common and in the females it's the ditch type.

3). The prevalence and distribution of FHNL is ethnic origin-independent.

4). The prevalence of the tongue type lesion increase with age while that of the ditch type decrease.

4.2. Femoral metrical/angular characteristics and FHNL

4.2.1. General population.

The relationship between FHNL and femur size and shape is presented in Table 4.2.1. Below we summarize the main findings:

1. Individuals with tongue or ditch lesions had significantly longer femurs (447.02 mm and 452.88 mm, respectively) than individuals with no lesions (438.50 mm). No significant difference in femoral length was found between individuals with ditch or tongue lesion.

84

2. Individuals with the ditch lesion manifested a significantly greater femoral trochanteric length (430.20 mm) compared to the no lesion group (418.92 mm) and the tongue type group (426.56 mm).

3. Maximum femoral neck length was significantly greater in the ditch group (96.28 mm) and tongue group (96.93 mm) compared to the no lesion group (92.98 mm). No difference was found in this parameter between the ditch group and the tongue group.

4. Minimum femoral neck length was significantly greater in the ditch group (85.10 mm) and tongue group (88.14 mm) compared to the no lesion group (82.54 mm). The tongue group had significantly greater minimum femoral neck length compared to the ditch group.

5. Femoral neck-shaft angle was significantly greater in the ditch type (128.93^0) compared to the tongue group (125.65^0) and the no lesion group (126.48^0).

6. No significant differences were found in torsion degree and shaft bowing angle between the three groups (ditch, tongue and no lesion).

4.2.2. Femoral metrical/angular characteristics and FHNL, males only.

The data for the males is presented in Table 4.2.2. The main findings were as follows:

1. Individuals with the ditch lesion had significantly longer femur (466.51 mm) than individuals with no lesions (454.89 mm). The ditch and tongue groups were similar with regard to femoral length.

2. No significant differences were found in greater trochanteric length between the three groups, although the ditch group showed a tendency to greater trochanteric length.

3. Maximum femoral neck length was significantly greater in the ditch (100.93 mm) and tongue groups (100.34 mm) compared to the no lesion group (97.54 mm). No difference was found in this parameter between the ditch and the tongue groups.

4. Minimum femoral neck length was significantly greater in the tongue group (91.36 mm) compared to the no lesion group (87.75 mm). No significant difference in minimum femoral neck length was found between individuals with tongue and ditch lesions (90.26 mm).

5. Femoral neck shaft angle was significantly greater in the ditch group (128.19^0) compared to the tongue group (125.74^0) and the no lesion group (126.48^0). It is interesting to note that the tongue group had the smallest neck-shaft angle.

6. Femoral torsion was similar in all three groups: the no lesion group (13.43 mm), the ditch group (10.98 mm) and the tongue group (11.59 mm). Similarly, no significant differences between the three groups were found in the bowing angle of the femoral shaft.

4.2.3. Femoral metrical/angular characteristics and FHNL, females only.

The data for the female population is presented in Table 4.2.3. The main findings were:

1. Individuals with the ditch lesion had significantly longer femurs (435.63 mm) than individuals with no lesion (422.11mm) or tongue lesion (421.51 mm).

2. Femoral greater trochanteric length was significantly greater in the ditch group (412.60 mm) compared to the tongue group (399.29 mm).

3. Femoral neck length was similar in all three groups.

4. Femoral neck-shaft angle was significantly greater in the ditch group (129.87^0) compared to the tongue (125.43^0) and the no lesion groups (125.76^0).

5. Femoral torsion was similar in the three groups.

6. Femoral shaft bowing angle was similar in the three groups.

4.2.4. Femoral metrical/angular characteristics and FHNL, European American samples.

The relationship between femoral size and shape and FHNL in the European American population is presented in Table 4.2.4. The main findings are presented below:

1. Individuals with the ditch lesion had significantly longer femurs (450.04mm) than individuals with no lesion (432.97 mm). No significant difference in femoral length was found between individuals with both the ditch and the tongue lesions (440.30mm).

2. Femoral greater trochanteric length was significantly greater in the ditch type group (428.07 mm) compared to the no lesion group (415.06 mm).

3. Maximum femoral neck length was significantly greater in the ditch (98.37 mm) and tongue groups (97.01 mm), compared to the no lesion group (91.99 mm). No significant difference was found in this parameter between the ditch and the tongue groups.

4. Minimum femoral neck length was significantly greater in the tongue group (89.24 mm) and the ditch group (88.92 mm) compared to the no lesion group (83.39 mm). No significant difference was found in this parameter between the tongue and the ditch groups.

5. Neck-shaft angle was similar in all three groups.

6. Femoral torsion was similar in all three groups.

7. Femoral shaft bowing angle was similar in all three groups.

4.2.5. Femoral metrical/angular characteristics and FHNL, African American samples.

The relationship between femoral size and shape and FHNL in African Americans is given in Table 4.2.5. The main findings were as follows:

1. Individuals with the tongue (457.25 mm) and ditch lesions (455.43 mm) had significantly longer femurs than individuals with no lesion (443.88 mm). No significant difference in femoral length was found between individuals with ditch and tongue lesion.

2. Femoral greater trochanteric length was significantly greater in the tongue group (436.67 mm) compared to the no lesion group (422.68 mm). No significant difference was found between the tongue and the ditch groups.

3. Maximum femoral neck length was similar in all three groups.

4. Minimum femoral neck length was significantly greater in the tongue group (86.48 mm) compared to the no lesion group (81.71 mm). Significant difference was also found between the tongue and the ditch group.

5. Femoral neck-shaft angle was significantly greater in the ditch group (130.27^0) compared to the tongue (126.27^0) and the no lesion group (127.46^0).

6. Femoral torsion was similar in all three groups.

7. Femoral shaft bowing angle was similar in all three groups.

4.2.6. Femoral metrical/angular characteristics and FHNL, European American males.

The relationship between femoral size and shape and FHNL in European American males appears in Table 4.2.6. The main findings were:

1. Individuals with the ditch lesion had significantly longer femur (463.55 mm) than individuals with no lesion (448.61 mm) or tongue (450.59 mm).

2. No significant difference in greater trochanteric length between the three groups was found.

3. Maximum femoral neck length was significantly greater in the ditch (102.20 mm) and the tongue groups (100.14 mm) compared to the no lesion group (96.83 mm). No significant difference was found in this parameter between the ditch and the tongue groups.

4. Minimum femoral neck length was significantly greater in the tongue (92.73 mm) and the ditch groups (92.41 mm) compared to the no lesion group (88.81 mm). No significant difference was found in this parameter between the tongue and the ditch groups.

5. No significant differences in neck-shaft angle, femoral torsion and femoral shaft bowing angle were found between the three groups.

4.2.7. Femoral metrical/angular characteristics and FHNL, African American males.

The relationship between femoral size and shape and FHNL in African American males appears in Table 4.2.7. The main findings were:

In all but one of the eight parameters, all three groups manifested similar values. The femoral torsion (bottom) was significantly smaller in the ditch group (10.78 mm) compared to the no lesion (14.74 mm) and the tongue groups (12.91 mm).

4.2.8. Femoral metrical/angular characteristics and FHNL, European American females.

The relationship between femoral size and shape and FHNL in European American females appears in Table 4.2.8. The main findings were:

1. Femoral length and femoral greater trochanteric length were similar in the three groups studied.

2. Maximum femoral neck length was significantly greater in the ditch group (91.63 mm) compared to the no lesion group (86.85 mm). No significant difference was found in this parameter between the ditch and the tongue group.

3. Minimum femoral neck length was significantly greater in the ditch group (81.79 mm) compared to the no lesion group (77.65 mm). No significant difference was found in this parameter between the ditch and the tongue group (80.45 mm).

4. The remaining parameters (neck-shaft angle, femoral head torsion and femoral shaft bowing angle), did not vary significantly between the three groups.

4.2.9. Femoral metrical/angular characteristics and FHNL, African American females.

The relationship between femoral size and shape and FHNL in African American females is given in Table 4.2.9. The main findings were:

1. Individuals with the ditch group had significantly longer femurs (442.82 mm) than individuals with no lesion (427.35 mm). No significant difference was found in femoral length between individuals with ditch or tongue lesion.

2. Femoral greater trochanteric length did not show significant differences between the three groups.

3. Maximum and minimum femoral neck length was similar in the three groups.

4. Femoral neck shaft-angle was significantly greater in the ditch group (131.05^{0}) compared to the tongue (124.60^{0}) or no lesion groups (124.65^{0}). No significant differences were detected between the tongue and the no lesion group.

5. The remaining parameters (neck-shaft angle, femoral head torsion and femoral shaft bowing angle), did not vary significantly between the three groups.

Table 4.2.1. Femoral metrical and angular characteristics by FHNL, general population.

Measurement	Lesions group	N	Mean	SD	P Value No lesion	Tongue
Femoral anatomical length	No lesion	142	438.50	28.34		
	Tongue	169	447.02	32.19	**0.051**	
	Ditch	154	452.88	30.67	**P<0.001**	0.229
Femoral greater trochanteric length	No lesion	142	418.92	27.12		
	Tongue	169	426.56	32.30	0.083	
	Ditch	154	430.20	29.78	**0.006**	0.551
Maximum femoral neck length	No lesion	142	92.98	7.66		
	Tongue	169	96.93	8.05	**P<0.001**	
	Ditch	154	96.28	7.95	**0.002**	0.758
Minimum femoral neck length	No lesion	142	82.54	7.74		
	Tongue	169	88.14	9.25	**P<0.001**	
	Ditch	154	85.10	8.89	**0.042**	**0.008**
Femoral neck-shaft angle	No lesion	142	126.48	5.40		
	Tongue	169	125.65	7.54	0.531	
	Ditch	154	128.93	6.04	**0.005**	**P<0.001**
Femoral torsion top	No lesion	142	57.02	8.14		
	Tongue	169	56.47	8.09	0.825	
	Ditch	154	55.30	7.54	0.232	0.510
Femoral torsion bottom	No lesion	142	12.61	5.87		
	Tongue	169	11.17	5.86	0.098	
	Ditch	154	10.85	5.65	0.677	0.647
Femoral shaft bowing angle	No lesion	142	158.39	2.22		
	Tongue	169	158.51	2.13	0.880	
	Ditch	154	158.87	2.16	0.161	0.334

Table 4.2.2. Femoral metrical and angular characteristics by FHNL, males only.

Measurement			Males only			
					P Value	
	Lesions group	N	Mean	SD	No lesion	Tongue
Femoral anatomical length	No lesion	71	454.89	23.99		
	Tongue	120	457.44	27.54	0.816	
	Ditch	86	466.51	27.73	**0.027**	0.058
Femoral greater trochanteric length	No lesion	71	434.17	22.09		
	Tongue	120	437.69	26.69	0.653	
	Ditch	86	444.12	26.22	0.053	0.204
Maximum femoral neck length	No lesion	71	97.54	5.71		
	Tongue	120	100.34	5.97	**0.007**	
	Ditch	86	100.93	6.30	**0.002**	0.789
Minimum femoral neck length	No lesion	71	87.75	5.88		
	Tongue	120	91.36	6.87	**0.002**	
	Ditch	86	90.26	6.89	0.064	0.503
Femoral neck shaft angle	No lesion	71	127.20	5.02		
	Tongue	120	125.74	6.19	0.254	
	Ditch	86	128.19	5.99	0.575	**0.014**
Femoral torsion top	No lesion	71	60.70	7.72		
	Tongue	120	58.68	7.59	0.201	
	Ditch	86	57.99	7.21	0.081	0.807
Femoral torsion bottom	No lesion	71	13.43	6.30		
	Tongue	120	11.59	6.20	0.147	
	Ditch	86	10.98	6.15	0.052	0.786
Femoral shaft bowing angle	No lesion	71	158.01	2.15		
	Tongue	120	158.49	2.10	0.293	
	Ditch	86	158.66	1.91	0.151	0.860

Table 4.2.3. Femoral metrical and angular characteristics by FHNL, females only.

Measurement	Females only					
					P Value	
	Lesions group	N	Mean	SD	No lesion	Tongue
Femoral anatomical length	No lesion	71	422.11	22.30		
	Tongue	49	421.51	28.46	0.999	
	Ditch	68	435.63	25.16	**0.007**	**0.012**
Femoral greater trochanteric length	No lesion	71	403.68	22.84		
	Tongue	49	399.29	28.57	0.639	
	Ditch	68	412.60	24.30	0.111	**0.019**
Maximum femoral neck length	No lesion	71	88.42	6.58		
	Tongue	49	88.47	5.94	0.999	
	Ditch	68	90.34	5.46	0.177	0.258
Minimum femoral neck length	No lesion	71	77.32	5.57		
	Tongue	49	80.27	9.67	0.091	
	Ditch	68	78.57	6.56	0.592	0.456
Femoral neck-shaft angle	No lesion	71	125.76	5.70		
	Tongue	49	125.43	10.18	0.970	
	Ditch	68	129.87	6.01	**0.004**	**0.005**
Femoral torsion top	No lesion	71	53.34	6.82		
	Tongue	49	51.04	6.64	0.188	
	Ditch	68	52.22	6.70	0.620	0.646
Femoral torsion bottom	No lesion	71	11.80	5.33		
	Tongue	49	10.16	4.86	0.225	
	Ditch	68	10.69	4.98	0.438	0.858
Femoral shaft bowing angle	No lesion	71	158.77	2.24		
	Tongue	49	158.56	2.23	0.888	
	Ditch	68	159.15	2.41	0.626	0.398

Table 4.2.4. Femoral metrical and angular characteristics by FHNL, European American only.

Measurement						P Value	
			European American only				
	Lesions group	N	Mean	SD	No lesion	Tongue
Femoral anatomical length	No lesion	70	432.97	27.57		
	Tongue	102	440.30	30.25	0.316	
	Ditch	73	450.04	35.02	**0.005**	0.126
Femoral greater trochanteric length	No lesion	70	415.06	26.53		
	Tongue	102	419.91	30.53	0.591	
	Ditch	73	428.07	33.65	**0.040**	0.219
Maximum femoral neck length	No lesion	70	91.99	7.13		
	Tongue	102	97.01	7.55	**P<0.001**	
	Ditch	73	98.73	8.30	**P<0.001**	0.347
Minimum femoral neck length	No lesion	70	83.39	7.66		
	Tongue	102	89.24	8.14	**P<0.001**	
	Ditch	73	88.92	8.48	**P<0.001**	0.968
Femoral neck-shaft angle	No lesion	70	125.47	5.90		
	Tongue	102	125.25	6.32	0.973	
	Ditch	73	127.44	6.47	0.173	0.075
Femoral torsion top	No lesion	70	55.96	8.14		
	Tongue	102	56.06	7.56	0.997	
	Ditch	73	55.56	7.99	0.956	0.918
Femoral torsion bottom	No lesion	70	11.68	5.52		
	Tongue	102	10.65	5.47	0.505	
	Ditch	73	10.34	6.04	0.373	0.940
Femoral shaft bowing angle	No lesion	70	157.75	1.92		
	Tongue	102	157.84	1.93	0.960	
	Ditch	73	157.97	2.25	0.819	0.923

Table 4.2.5. Femoral metrical and angular characteristics by FHNL, African American only.

| Measurement | African American only | | | | | |
| | Lesions group | N | Mean | SD | P Value | |
					No lesion	Tongue
Femoral anatomical length	No lesion	72	443.88	28.23		
	Tongue	67	457.25	32.56	**0.026**	
	Ditch	81	455.43	26.10	**0.049**	0.930
Femoral greater trochanteric length	No lesion	72	422.68	27.33		
	Tongue	67	436.67	32.52	**0.017**	
	Ditch	81	432.12	25.87	0.126	0.113
Maximum femoral neck length	No lesion	72	93.94	8.06		
	Tongue	67	96.82	8.80	0.104	
	Ditch	81	94.07	6.96	0.995	0.113
Minimum femoral neck length	No lesion	72	81.71	7.78		
	Tongue	67	86.48	10.58	**0.006**	
	Ditch	81	81.65	7.83	0.999	**0.004**
Femoral neck-shaft angle	No lesion	72	127.46	4.70		
	Tongue	67	126.27	9.10	0.565	
	Ditch	81	130.27	5.31	**0.031**	**0.001**
Femoral torsion top	No lesion	72	58.06	8.07		
	Tongue	67	57.09	8.86	0.777	
	Ditch	81	58.33	7.15	0.113	0.416
Femoral torsion bottom	No lesion	72	13.51	6.08		
	Tongue	67	11.98	6.38	0.322	
	Ditch	81	11.31	5.27	0.074	0.787
Femoral shaft bowing angle	No lesion	72	159.01	2.34		
	Tongue	67	159.53	2.04	0.313	
	Ditch	81	159.69	1.71	0.120	0.901

Table 4.2.6. Femoral metrical and angular characteristics by FHNL, European American males only.

Measurement	European American males only					
	Lesions group	N	Mean	SD	P Value	
					No lesion	Tongue
Femoral anatomical length	No lesion	36	448.61	26.20		
	Tongue	73	450.59	23.93	0.937	
	Ditch	49	463.55	31.54	**0.044**	**0.037**
Femoral greater trochanteric length	No lesion	36	428.75	23.99		
	Tongue	73	431.18	22.69	0.895	
	Ditch	49	441.71	29.41	0.068	0.081
Maximum femoral neck length	No lesion	36	96.83	5.46		
	Tongue	73	100.14	5.37	**0.033**	
	Ditch	49	102.20	7.24	**0.001**	0.193
Minimum femoral neck length	No lesion	36	88.81	5.43		
	Tongue	73	92.73	5.68	**0.008**	
	Ditch	49	92.41	7.09	**0.028**	0.961
Femoral neck-shaft angle	No lesion	36	126.11	5.50		
	Tongue	73	124.95	6.33	0.658	
	Ditch	49	127.31	6.62	0.685	0.127
Femoral torsion top	No lesion	36	59.50	7.81		
	Tongue	73	57.81	7	0.524	
	Ditch	49	58.16	7.30	0.706	0.966
Femoral torsion bottom	No lesion	36	12.17	5.98		
	Tongue	73	10.75	5.60	0.512	
	Ditch	49	11.12	6.40	0.729	0.945
Femoral shaft bowing angle	No lesion	36	157.47	1.95		
	Tongue	73	157.89	1.87	0.555	
	Ditch	49	158.02	1.82	0.419	0.933

Table 4.2.7. Femoral metrical and angular characteristics by FHNL, African American males only.

Measurement	African American males only					
					P Value	
	Lesions group	N	Mean	SD	No lesion	Tongue
Femoral anatomical length	No lesion	35	461.34	19.85		
	Tongue	47	468.09	29.59	0.474	
	Ditch	37	470.43	21.98	0.297	0.910
Femoral greater trochanteric length	No lesion	35	439.74	18.69		
	Tongue	47	447.81	29.42	0.332	
	Ditch	37	447.30	21.25	0.419	0.995
Maximum femoral neck length	No lesion	35	98.26	5.43		
	Tongue	47	100.79	6.84	0.149	
	Ditch	37	99.35	4.37	0.724	0.527
Minimum Femoral neck length	No lesion	35	86.66	6.21		
	Tongue	47	89.32	8.02	0.244	
	Ditch	37	87.41	5.63	0.898	0.479
Femoral neck-shaft angle	No lesion	35	128.31	4.26		
	Tongue	47	126.98	5.83	0.508	
	Ditch	37	129.35	4.90	0.693	0.114
Femoral torsion top	No lesion	35	61.94	7.54		
	Tongue	47	60.04	8.32	0.550	
	Ditch	37	57.76	7.19	0.077	0.410
Femoral torsion bottom	No lesion	35	14.74	6.44		
	Tongue	47	12.91	6.90	0.463	
	Ditch	37	10.78	5.88	**0.040**	0.333
Femoral shaft bowing angle	No lesion	35	158.56	2.23		
	Tongue	47	159.44	2.11	0.162	
	Ditch	37	159.50	1.72	0.154	0.991

Table 4.2.8. Femoral metrical and angular characteristics by FHNL, European American females only.

Measurement	Lesions group	N	Mean	SD	P Value No lesion	P Value Tongue
Femoral anatomical length	No lesion	34	416.41	17.65		
	Tongue	29	414.41	29.31	0.947	
	Ditch	24	422.46	24.13	0.638	0.477
Femoral greater trochanteric length	No lesion	34	400.56	21		
	Tongue	29	391.55	29.56	0.358	
	Ditch	24	400.21	23.09	0.999	0.450
Maximum femoral neck length	No lesion	34	86.85	4		
	Tongue	29	89.14	6.49	0.239	
	Ditch	24	91.63	5.30	**0.005**	0.241
Minimum femoral neck length	No lesion	34	77.65	5.04		
	Tongue	29	80.45	6.66	0.193	
	Ditch	24	81.79	6.56	**0.042**	0.724
Femoral neck-shaft angle	No lesion	34	124.79	6.30		
	Tongue	29	126	6.35	0.753	
	Ditch	24	127.71	6.29	0.230	0.621
Femoral torsion top	No lesion	34	52.21	6.75		
	Tongue	29	51.66	7.22	0.951	
	Ditch	24	50.25	6.68	0.570	0.762
Femoral torsion bottom	No lesion	34	11.18	5.05		
	Tongue	29	10.38	5.20	0.825	
	Ditch	24	8.75	4.96	0.207	0.512
Femoral shaft bowing angle	No lesion	34	158.05	1.86		
	Tongue	29	157.73	2.09	0.858	
	Ditch	24	157.86	2.98	0.955	0.977

Table 4.2.9. Femoral metrical and angular characteristics by FHNL, African American females only.

Measurement	African American females only					
	Lesions group	N	Mean	SD	P Value	
					No lesion	Tongue
Femoral anatomical length	No lesion	37	427.35	24.95		
	Tongue	20	431.80	24.32	0.800	
	Ditch	44	442.82	22.91	**0.018**	0.239
Femoral greater trochanteric length	No lesion	37	406.54	24.34		
	Tongue	20	410.50	23.48	0.830	
	Ditch	44	419.36	22.42	0.053	0.375
Maximum femoral neck length	No lesion	37	89.86	8.08		
	Tongue	20	87.50	5.05	0.425	
	Ditch	44	89.64	5.47	0.988	0.477
Minimum femoral neck length	No lesion	37	77.03	6.06		
	Tongue	20	80	13.06	0.400	
	Ditch	44	76.82	5.93	0.993	0.330
Femoral neck-shaft angle	No lesion	37	124.65	5		
	Tongue	20	124.60	14.19	0.645	
	Ditch	44	131.05	5.57	**0.048**	**0.012**
Femoral torsion top	No lesion	37	54.38	6.80		
	Tongue	20	50.15	5.76	0.069	
	Ditch	44	53.30	6.53	0.757	0.205
Femoral torsion bottom	No lesion	37	12.38	5.58		
	Tongue	20	9.85	4.42	0.196	
	Ditch	44	11.75	4.72	0.854	0.375
Femoral shaft bowing angle	No lesion	37	159.43	2.39		
	Tongue	20	159.76	1.90	0.836	
	Ditch	44	159.85	1.70	0.648	0.988

4.3. Pelvic metrical/angular characteristics and FHNL

4.3.1. Pelvic metrical/angular characteristics and FHNL, general population.

The relationship between pelvic size and shape and FHNL in the general population is presented in Table 4.3.1. The main findings were:

None of the pelvic parameters in the three groups studied were significantly different, except for the sacral inclination angle, which was significantly greater in individuals with the ditch lesion (51.18^0) compared to individuals with no lesion group (47.8^0). No significant difference was found in sacral inclination angle between individuals with ditch and tongue lesions.

4.3.2. Pelvic metrical/angular characteristics and FHNL, males only.

The relationship between pelvic size and shape and FHNL in males is presented in Table 4.3.2. The main findings were:

No significant differences were found between the three groups in all pelvic parameters.

4.3.3. Pelvic metrical/angular characteristics and FHNL, females only.

The relationship between pelvic size and shape and FHNL in females is presented in Table 4.3.3. The main findings were:

No significant differences in size and shape of the pelvis between the three groups studied were found.

4.3.4. Pelvic metrical/angular characteristics and FHNL, European American samples.

The relationship between pelvic size and shape and FHNL in European American are presented in Table 4.3.4. Below we summarize the main findings:

No significant differences in pelvic parameters were found between the three groups.

4.3.5. Pelvic metrical/angular characteristics and FHNL, African American samples.

The relationship between pelvic size and shape and FHNL in African Americans is presented in Table 4.3.5. Below we summarize the main findings:

None of the parameters in the three groups were significantly different, except for the sacral inclination angle, which was significantly greater in individuals with the ditch lesion (50.29^0) compared to individuals with no lesion (45.48^0). No significant difference was found in sacral inclination angle between individuals with ditch and tongue lesions.

4.3.6. Pelvic metrical/angular characteristics and FHNL, European American males.

The relationship between pelvic size and shape and FHNL in European American males is presented in Table 4.3.6. Below we summarize the main findings:

No significant differences in pelvic parameters were found between the three groups studied.

4.3.7. Pelvic metrical/angular characteristics and FHNL, African American males.

The relationship between pelvic size and shape and FHNL in African American males is presented in Table 4.3.7. Below we summarize the main findings:

No significant differences in all pelvic parameters were found between the three groups studied.

4.3.8. Pelvic metrical/angular characteristics and FHNL, European American females.

None of the parameters in the three groups were significantly different, except for ischial tuberosity width, which was significantly greater in individuals with the tongue lesion (133.90 mm) compared to individuals with no lesion (124.07 mm). No significant difference was found in ischial tuberosity width between individuals with tongue and ditch lesions (Table 4.3.8).

4.3.9. Pelvic metrical/angular characteristics and FHNL, African American females.

The relationship between pelvic size and shape and FHNL in African American females is presented in Table 4.3.9. The main findings were:

None of the parameters in the three groups were significantly different, except for the sacral inclination angle, which was significantly greater in individuals with the ditch lesion (51.21^0) compared to individuals with no lesion (44.44^0). No significant difference was found in sacral inclination angle between individuals with ditch and tongue lesions.

Table 4.3.1. Pelvic metrical and angular characteristics by FHNL, general population.

Measurement	Lesions group	N	Mean	SD	P Value	
					No lesion	Tongue
Posterior superior iliac spine width	No lesion	115	78.41	9.62		
	Tongue	133	77.46	9.63	0.736	
	Ditch	120	78.76	9.22	0.961	0.555
Schiatic notch width	No lesion	115	135.56	8.95		
	Tongue	133	136.56	9.51	0.720	
	Ditch	120	173.17	10.39	0.446	0.883
Ischial spine width	No lesion	115	101.39	12.29		
	Tongue	133	100.38	11.86	0.803	
	Ditch	120	100.77	11.77	0.926	0.966
Ischial tuberosity width	No lesion	115	117.21	12.39		
	Tongue	133	119.23	15.20	0.538	
	Ditch	120	121.13	14.74	0.110	0.572
Anterior superior iliac spine width	No lesion	115	223.23	19.54		
	Tongue	133	226.23	20.70	0.510	
	Ditch	120	224.67	20.55	0.862	0.830
Left ASIS Left PSIS width	No lesion	115	149.46	10.48		
	Tongue	133	151.26	9.76	0.365	
	Ditch	120	151.58	9.48	0.265	0.968
Sacral inclination angle	No lesion	115	47.80	10.93		
	Tongue	133	49.11	10.20	0.614	
	Ditch	120	51.18	9.96	**0.046**	0.285
Pelvic width	No lesion	115	264	20.14		
	Tongue	133	268.77	22.39	0.216	
	Ditch	120	266.53	21.06	0.663	0.705
Pelvic height	No lesion	115	202	14.64		
	Tongue	133	205.84	13.89	0.105	
	Ditch	120	204.68	13.99	0.350	0.810

Table 4.3.2. Pelvic metrical and angular characteristics by FHNL, males only.

| Measurement | Males only | | | | P Value | |
	Lesions group	N	Mean	SD	No lesion	Tongue
Posterior superior iliac spine width	No lesion	61	74.46	8.34		
	Tongue	92	76.23	9.52	0.477	
	Ditch	70	76.33	8.20	0.481	0.998
Schiatic notch width	No lesion	61	132.83	9.40		
	Tongue	92	136.12	8.98	0.110	
	Ditch	70	136.64	10.0	0.072	0.942
Ischial spine width	No lesion	61	92.84	8.98		
	Tongue	92	96.06	8.73	0.081	
	Ditch	70	94.48	8.25	0.555	0.519
Ischial tuberosity width	No lesion	61	110.40	10.29		
	Tongue	92	113.86	11.45	0.202	
	Ditch	70	114.74	12.96	0.107	0.893
Anterior superior iliac spine width	No lesion	61	225.96	19.40		
	Tongue	92	229.36	19.03	0.573	
	Ditch	70	228.16	20.19	0.813	0.927
Left ASIS Left PSIS width	No lesion	61	152.77	9.89		
	Tongue	92	152.79	9.09	1.000	
	Ditch	70	154.02	9.24	0.745	0.710
Sacral inclination angle	No lesion	61	47.79	9.79		
	Tongue	92	48.88	10.54	0.810	
	Ditch	70	51	10.06	0.200	0.424
Pelvic width	No lesion	61	265.88	19.17		
	Tongue	92	272.61	21.57	0.147	
	Ditch	70	269.87	20.50	0.547	0.705
Pelvic height	No lesion	61	210.49	13.06		
	Tongue	92	211.05	11.30	0.960	
	Ditch	70	211.67	11.50	0.851	0.948

Table 4.3.3. Pelvic metrical and angular characteristics by FHNL, females only.

Measurement	Females only				P Value	
	Lesions group	N	Mean	SD	No lesion	Tongue
Posterior superior iliac spine width	No lesion	54	82.87	9.06		
	Tongue	41	80.22	9.43	0.394	
	Ditch	50	82.17	9.58	0.928	0.615
Schiatic notch width	No lesion	54	138.65	7.36		
	Tongue	41	137.54	10.66	0.859	
	Ditch	50	137.90	10.97	0.926	0.985
Ischial spine width	No lesion	54	111.05	7.38		
	Tongue	41	110.07	12.31	0.894	
	Ditch	50	109.58	10.25	0.755	0.973
Ischial tuberosity width	No lesion	54	124.90	9.84		
	Tongue	41	131.29	15.77	0.053	
	Ditch	50	130.07	12.29	0.116	0.900
Anterior superior iliac spine width	No lesion	54	220.14	19.42		
	Tongue	41	219.20	22.74	0.976	
	Ditch	50	219.79	20.25	0.996	0.991
Left ASIS Left PSIS width	No lesion	54	145.73	9.95		
	Tongue	41	147.81	10.44	0.587	
	Ditch	50	148.15	8.80	0.451	0.987
Sacral inclination angle	No lesion	54	47.82	12.17		
	Tongue	41	49.62	9.51	0.722	
	Ditch	50	51.42	9.91	0.234	0.726
Pelvic width	No lesion	54	261.91	21.16		
	Tongue	41	260.15	22.06	0.924	
	Ditch	50	261.84	21.13	1.000	0.932
Pelvic height	No lesion	54	192.41	9.56		
	Tongue	41	194.15	11.98	0.739	
	Ditch	50	194.90	11.02	0.502	0.947

Table 4.3.4. Pelvic metrical and angular characteristics by FHNL, European American only.

| Measurement | European American only | | | | P Value | |
	Lesions group	N	Mean	SD	No lesion	Tongue
Posterior superior iliac spine width	No lesion	56	80.08	8.36		
	Tongue	80	79.71	9.56	0.973	
	Ditch	59	80.20	9.07	0.998	0.953
Schiatic notch width	No lesion	56	139.56	8.52		
	Tongue	80	140.15	7.99	0.927	
	Ditch	59	141.81	9.75	0.388	0.544
Ischial spine width	No lesion	56	101.86	12.63		
	Tongue	80	102.86	11.54	0.886	
	Ditch	59	100.80	10.61	0.887	0.588
Ischial tuberosity width	No lesion	56	117.90	11.98		
	Tongue	80	122.19	15.07	0.197	
	Ditch	59	122.80	12.99	0.159	0.967
Anterior superior iliac spine width	No lesion	56	231.52	19.38		
	Tongue	80	231.90	18.39	0.994	
	Ditch	59	234.22	20.25	0.754	0.781
Left ASIS Left PSIS width	No lesion	56	153.91	9.93		
	Tongue	80	153.82	8.43	0.998	
	Ditch	59	155.98	8.91	0.471	0.379
Sacral inclination angle	No lesion	56	50.43	10.79		
	Tongue	80	49.96	10.24	0.966	
	Ditch	59	52.09	10.04	0.691	0.487
Pelvic width	No lesion	56	275.76	17.27		
	Tongue	80	276.33	19.49	0.986	
	Ditch	59	277.68	19.79	0.865	0.917
Pelvic height	No lesion	56	204.98	15.34		
	Tongue	80	207.60	13.28	0.556	
	Ditch	59	211.15	13.10	0.060	0.329

Table 4.3.5. Pelvic metrical and angular characteristics by FHNL, African American only.

| Measurement | African American only | | | | P Value | |
	Lesions group	N	Mean	SD	No lesion	Tongue
Posterior superior iliac spine width	No lesion	58	76.75	10.59		
	Tongue	53	74.06	8.78	0.340	
	Ditch	61	77.37	9.23	0.939	0.188
Schiatic notch width	No lesion	58	131.49	7.41		
	Tongue	53	131.13	9.09	0.976	
	Ditch	61	132.68	8.98	0.751	0.630
Ischial spine width	No lesion	58	101	12.15		
	Tongue	53	96.64	11.44	0.173	
	Ditch	61	100.75	12.89	0.993	0.204
Ischial tuberosity width	No lesion	58	116.59	12.95		
	Tongue	53	114.76	14.40	0.808	
	Ditch	61	119.51	16.20	0.553	0.227
Anterior superior iliac spine width	No lesion	58	214.50	15.01		
	Tongue	53	217.68	21.22	0.636	
	Ditch	61	215.44	16.28	0.958	0.794
Left ASIS Left PSIS width	No lesion	58	144.68	8.24		
	Tongue	53	147.40	10.43	0.278	
	Ditch	61	147.32	8.01	0.275	0.999
Sacral inclination angle	No lesion	58	45.48	10.56		
	Tongue	53	47.82	10.11	0.481	
	Ditch	61	50.29	9.88	**0.038**	0.436
Pelvic width	No lesion	58	252.28	15.15		
	Tongue	53	257.36	21.80	0.325	
	Ditch	61	255.74	16.13	0.570	0.889
Pelvic height	No lesion	58	198.52	12.62		
	Tongue	53	203.19	14.49	0.170	
	Ditch	61	198.43	11.88	0.999	0.151

Table 4.3.6. Pelvic metrical and angular characteristics by FHNL, European American males only.

Measurement	European American males only				P Value	
	Lesions group	N	Mean	SD	No lesion	Tongue
Posterior superior iliac spine width	No lesion	30	78.06	7.88		
	Tongue	55	78.36	9.55	0.950	
	Ditch	42	78.44	8.50	0.990	0.982
Schiatic notch width	No lesion	30	137.25	9.04		
	Tongue	55	139.77	8.05	0.452	
	Ditch	42	140.97	9.50	0.212	0.800
Ischial spine width	No lesion	30	94.11	10.40		
	Tongue	55	98.39	8.77	0.107	
	Ditch	42	96.47	7.67	0.539	0.571
Ischial tuberosity width	No lesion	30	112.55	10.67		
	Tongue	55	116.87	11.66	0.249	
	Ditch	42	118.68	11.42	0.082	0.741
Anterior superior iliac spine width	No lesion	30	235.05	17.33		
	Tongue	55	235.94	17.25	0.977	
	Ditch	42	235.14	19.64	1.000	0.977
Left ASIS Left PSIS width	No lesion	30	156.27	9.96		
	Tongue	55	155.38	8.40	0.909	
	Ditch	42	157.23	8.98	0.904	0.602
Sacral inclination angle	No lesion	30	49.53	9.14		
	Tongue	55	49.75	10.91	0.955	
	Ditch	42	52.20	9.92	0.552	0.506
Pelvic width	No lesion	30	275.90	16.59		
	Tongue	55	280.58	19.22	0.555	
	Ditch	42	278.12	19.57	0.887	0.815
Pelvic height	No lesion	30	213.50	14.30		
	Tongue	55	213.18	11.08	0.993	
	Ditch	42	216.10	10.83	0.658	0.488

Table 4.3.7. Pelvic metrical and angular characteristics by FHNL, African American males only.

| Measurement | African American males only | | | | P Value | |
	Lesions group	N	Mean	SD	No lesion	Tongue
Posterior superior iliac spine width	No lesion	30	70.64	7.21		
	Tongue	37	72.55	8.30	0.588	
	Ditch	28	73.28	6.79	0.414	0.928
Schiatic notch width	No lesion	30	127.92	6.94		
	Tongue	37	130.71	7.49	0.286	
	Ditch	28	130.14	6.77	0.497	0.951
Ischial spine width	No lesion	30	91.42	7.36		
	Tongue	37	92.59	7.53	0.826	
	Ditch	28	91.51	8.34	0.999	0.855
Ischial tuberosity width	No lesion	30	108.11	9.72		
	Tongue	37	109.38	9.64	0.891	
	Ditch	28	108.84	13.08	0.968	0.980
Anterior superior iliac spine width	No lesion	30	215.56	15.10		
	Tongue	37	219.59	17.46	0.609	
	Ditch	28	217.68	16.32	0.887	0.898
Left ASIS Left PSIS width	No lesion	30	148.42	7.01		
	Tongue	37	148.95	8.80	0.964	
	Ditch	28	149.21	7.47	0.931	0.992
Sacral inclination angle	No lesion	30	46.44	10.24		
	Tongue	37	47.58	9.96	0.901	
	Ditch	28	49.20	10.16	0.585	0.815
Pelvic width	No lesion	30	255.17	15.13		
	Tongue	37	260.76	19.50	0.411	
	Ditch	28	257.50	15.11	0.872	0.747
Pelvic height	No lesion	30	206.60	9.96		
	Tongue	37	207.89	11.02	0.875	
	Ditch	28	205.04	9.15	0.843	0.536

Table 4.3.8. Pelvic metrical and angular characteristics by FHNL, European American females only.

| Measurement | European American females only | | | | P Value | |
	Lesions group	N	Mean	SD	No lesion	Tongue
Posterior superior iliac spine width	No lesion	26	82.42	8.43		
	Tongue	25	81.92	9.40	0.981	
	Ditch	17	84.74	9.08	0.710	0.610
Schiatic notch width	No lesion	26	142.24	7.15		
	Tongue	25	141.01	7.97	0.871	
	Ditch	17	143.87	10.35	0.821	0.554
Ischial spine width	No lesion	26	110.81	8.38		
	Tongue	25	112.68	10.93	0.786	
	Ditch	17	111.52	9.27	0.972	0.928
Ischial tuberosity width	No lesion	26	124.07	10.49		
	Tongue	25	133.90	15.30	**0.026**	
	Ditch	17	132.97	11.06	0.085	0.973
Anterior superior iliac spine width	No lesion	26	227.45	21.12		
	Tongue	25	223	17.99	0.737	
	Ditch	17	231.95	22.13	0.778	0.379
Left ASIS Left PSIS width	No lesion	26	151.18	9.34		
	Tongue	25	150.38	7.57	0.945	
	Ditch	17	152.88	8.16	0.813	0.644
Sacral inclination angle	No lesion	26	51.47	12.55		
	Tongue	25	50.41	8.77	0.941	
	Ditch	17	51.83	10.63	0.994	0.917
Pelvic width	No lesion	26	275.62	18.32		
	Tongue	25	266.96	16.94	0.255	
	Ditch	17	276.59	20.89	0.986	0.261
Pelvic height	No lesion	26	195.15	9.63		
	Tongue	25	195.32	8.70	0.998	
	Ditch	17	198.94	9.95	0.438	0.475

Table 4.3.9. Pelvic metrical and angular characteristics by FHNL, African American females only.

| Measurement | African American females only | | | | P Value | |
	Lesions group	N	Mean	SD	No lesion	Tongue
Posterior superior iliac spine width	No lesion	28	83.30	9.74		
	Tongue	16	77.56	9.12	0.169	
	Ditch	33	80.84	9.69	0.611	0.536
Schiatic notch width	No lesion	28	135.32	5.91		
	Tongue	16	132.12	12.26	0.555	
	Ditch	33	134.83	10.11	0.979	0.639
Ischial spine width	No lesion	28	111.28	6.47		
	Tongue	16	105.99	13.56	0.256	
	Ditch	33	108.58	10.71	0.587	0.703
Ischial tuberosity width	No lesion	28	125.68	9.33		
	Tongue	16	127.21	16.12	0.926	
	Ditch	33	128.57	12.79	0.666	0.937
Anterior superior iliac spine width	No lesion	28	213.35	15.12		
	Tongue	16	213.26	28.28	1.000	
	Ditch	33	213.53	16.26	0.999	0.999
Left ASIS Left PSIS width	No lesion	28	140.67	7.64		
	Tongue	16	143.80	13.08	0.560	
	Ditch	33	145.71	8.21	0.112	0.795
Sacral inclination angle	No lesion	28	44.44	10.98		
	Tongue	16	48.37	10.74	0.485	
	Ditch	33	51.21	9.69	**0.046**	0.670
Pelvic width	No lesion	28	249.18	14.81		
	Tongue	16	249.50	25.30	0.998	
	Ditch	33	254.24	17.03	0.563	0.698
Pelvic height	No lesion	28	189.86	8.92		
	Tongue	16	192.31	15.99	0.796	
	Ditch	33	192.82	11.10	0.612	0.990

4.4. Acetabular metrical and angular characteristics by FHNL

4.4.1. General population.

The relationship between acetabular size and shape and FHNL is presented in Table 4.4.1. Below we summarize the main findings.

1. Bi-acetabular depth distance and bi-acetabular rim distance were similar in all three groups studied.

2. Individuals with tongue lesions had significantly greater horizontal acetabular diameters (52.11mm) than individuals with no lesions (51.06 mm). No significant difference was found in horizontal acetabular diameter between individuals with ditch and tongue lesions.

3. Vertical acetabular diameter, acetabular inclination and version angle did not vary significantly between the three groups.

4. Acetabular depth was significantly greater in the ditch (22.97 mm) and the tongue groups (22.66 mm) compared to the no lesion group (21.88 mm). No significant difference was found between ditch and tongue groups.

4.4.2. Acetabular metrical and angular characteristics by FHNL, males only.

The relationship between acetabular size and shape and FHNL in males is presented in Table 4.4.2. Below we summarize the main findings:

1. Bi-acetabular depth distance, bi-acetabular rim distance, horizontal acetabular diameter and vertical acetabular diameter did not vary significantly among the three groups.

2. Individuals with tongue (65.23^0) or ditch lesions (63.90^0) had significantly smaller acetabular inclination angles than individuals with no lesion (67.45^0). No significant difference was found in the acetabular inclination angle between individuals with ditch and tongue lesions.

3. Acetabular version angle was similar in all three groups.

4. Acetabular depth was significantly greater in the ditch group (24.13 mm) than the no lesion group (23.13 mm). No significant difference was found between the tongue and the ditch group.

4.4.3. Acetabular metrical and angular characteristics by FHNL, females only.

The relationship between acetabular size and shape and FHNL in females is presented in Table 4.4.3. The main findings were:

1. Bi-acetabular depth distance, bi-acetabular rim distance, horizontal acetabular diameter, and vertical acetabular diameter did not vary significantly among the three groups.

2. Individuals with ditch (72.19^0) or tongue lesions (72.17^0) had significantly greater acetabular inclination angle than individuals in the no lesion group (68.50^0). No significant difference was found in the acetabular inclination angle between individuals with ditch and tongue lesions.

3. Individuals with ditch (48.49^0) or tongue (48.18^0) had significantly greater acetabular version angle than individuals with no lesion (44.72^0). No significant difference was found in acetabular version angle between individuals with ditch and tongue lesions.

4. Acetabular depth was significantly greater in the ditch group (21.96 mm) compared to the tongue (20.91 mm) or no lesion group (20.92). No significant difference was found between the tongue and the no lesion group.

4.4.4. Acetabular metrical and angular characteristics by FHNL, European American only.

The relationship between acetabular size and shape and FHNL in European American is presented in Table 4.4.4. The main findings were:

1. Bi-acetabular depth distance and bi-acetabular rim distance did not vary significantly between the three groups studied.

2. Individuals with the ditch lesion had significantly greater horizontal acetabular diameter (53.06 mm) than individuals with no lesion (50.96 mm). No significant difference was found in horizontal acetabular diameter between individuals with tongue or ditch.

3. Vertical acetabular diameter, acetabular inclination angle and acetabular version angle did not vary significantly among the three groups.

4. Acetabular depth was significantly greater in the ditch group (23.46 mm) compared to the no lesion (22.04 mm) or tongue group (22.91 mm). No significant difference was found between tongue and no lesion group.

4.4.5. Acetabular metrical and angular characteristics by FHNL, African American only.

The relationship between acetabular size and shape and FHNL in African American is presented in Table 4.4.5. The main findings were:

No differences in any of the seven parameters studied were found between the three groups.

4.4.6. Acetabular metrical and angular characteristics by FHNL, European American males only.

The relationship between acetabular size and shape and FHNL in European American males is presented in Table 4.4.6. The main findings were:

No differences were found between the three groups in the seven parameters of the pelvis.

4.4.7. Acetabular metrical and angular characteristics by FHNL, African American males only.

The relationship between acetabular size and shape and FHNL in African American males is presented in Table 4.4.7. The main findings were:

None of the parameters in the three groups were significantly different, except for the acetabular inclination angle, which was significantly smaller in individuals with tongue (65.04^{0}) or ditch lesions (63.92^{0}) compared to individuals with no lesion

(69.13^0). No significant difference in acetabular inclination angle between individuals with ditch and tongue lesions was found.

4.4.8. Acetabular metrical and angular characteristics by FHNL, European American females only.

The relationship between acetabular size and shape and FHNL in European American females is presented in Table 4.4.8. The main findings were:

1. Bi-acetabular depth distance, bi-acetabular rim distance, horizontal acetabular diameter and vertical acetabular diameter did not vary significantly among the three groups.

2. Individuals with ditch (72.05^0) or tongue lesions (70.98^0) had significantly greater acetabular inclination angles than individuals with no lesion (66.73^0). No significant difference was found in the acetabular inclination angle between individuals with ditch and tongue lesions.

3. Individuals with tongue (47.66^0) or ditch lesions (47.59^0) had significantly greater acetabular version angles than individuals with no lesion (43.71^0). No significant difference was found in the acetabular version angle between individuals with ditch and tongue lesions.

4.4.9. Acetabular metrical and angular characteristics by FHNL, African American females only.

The relationship between acetabular size and shape and FHNL in African American females is presented in Table 4.4.9. The main findings were:

1. Acetabular depth width, superior acetabular width, horizontal acetabular diameter, vertical acetabular diameter and acetabular inclination angle did not vary significantly among the three groups.

2. Individuals with ditch lesion (48.95^0) had significantly greater acetabular version angles than individuals with no lesion (45.66^0). No significant differences were found in acetabular version angle between individuals with tongue and ditch lesion.

114

3. Acetabular depth was significantly greater in the ditch group (22.12 mm) compared to tongue group (20.67mm). No significant difference was found between the ditch group and the no lesion groups.

Table 4.4.1. Acetabular metrical and angular characteristics by FHNL, general population.

Measurement	Lesions group	N	Mean	SD	P Value No lesion	Tongue
Bi-acetabular depth distance	No lesion	115	148.43	9.11		
	Tongue	133	148.21	9.60	0.985	
	Ditch	120	149.45	11.19	0.740	0.618
Bi-acetabular rim distance	No lesion	115	183.29	10.48		0.304
	Tongue	133	185.56	11.18	0.304	
	Ditch	120	185.39	12.84	0.378	0.993
Horizontal acetabular diameter	No lesion	115	51.06	4.24		
	Tongue	133	52.11	4.20	**0.011**	
	Ditch	120	51.67	3.98	0.242	0.432
Vertical acetabular diameter	No lesion	115	54.17	4.58		
	Tongue	133	54.30	3.83	0.988	
	Ditch	120	54.10	4.25	0.967	0.912
Acetabular inclination angle	No lesion	115	67.94	4.64		
	Tongue	133	67.37	6.22	0.748	
	Ditch	120	67.36	6.52	0.750	1.000
Acetabular version angle	No lesion	115	45.81	4.45		
	Tongue	133	46.81	4.66	0.229	
	Ditch	120	46.94	4.45	0.164	0.973
Acetabular depth	No lesion	115	21.88	1.99		
	Tongue	133	22.66	2.36	**0.021**	
	Ditch	120	22.97	2.20	**P<0.001**	0.538

Table 4.4.2. Acetabular metrical and angular characteristics by FHNL, males only.

Measurement	Males only				P Value	
	Lesions group	N	Mean	SD	No lesion	Tongue
Bi-acetabular depth distance	No lesion	61	146.37	9.30		
	Tongue	92	147.37	8.84	0.822	
	Ditch	70	148.90	11.08	0.332	0.612
Bi-acetabular rim distance	No lesion	61	184.69	10.68		
	Tongue	92	187.69	10.61	0.372	
	Ditch	70	187.70	12.80	0.321	0.980
Horizontal acetabular diameter	No lesion	61	53.77	3.35		
	Tongue	92	54.12	2.96	0.795	
	Ditch	70	53.90	3.15	0.971	0.909
Vertical acetabular diameter	No lesion	61	56.99	3.79		
	Tongue	92	55.76	2.93	0.082	
	Ditch	70	56.03	3.25	0.256	0.877
Acetabular inclination angle	No lesion	61	67.45	4.34		
	Tongue	92	65.23	5.03	**0.021**	
	Ditch	70	63.90	4.80	**P<0.001**	0.220
Acetabular version angle	No lesion	61	46.78	3.81		
	Tongue	92	46.20	4.59	0.721	
	Ditch	70	45.84	4.52	0.470	0.875
Acetabular depth	No lesion	61	23.13	1.91		
	Tongue	92	23.56	2.01	0.436	
	Ditch	70	24.13	2.03	**0.019**	0.201

Table 4.4.3. Acetabular metrical and angular characteristics by FHNL, females only.

| Measurement | Females only | | | | P Value | |
	Lesions group	N	Mean	SD	No lesion	Tongue
Bi-acetabular depth distance	No lesion	54	150.76	8.36		
	Tongue	41	150.08	11.02	0.950	
	Ditch	50	150.21	11.41	0.962	0.998
Bi-acetabular rim distance	No lesion	54	181.71	10.10		
	Tongue	41	181.58	11.53	0.999	
	Ditch	50	182.17	12.30	0.979	0.971
Horizontal acetabular diameter	No lesion	54	48.01	2.83		
	Tongue	41	47.62	2.89	0.801	
	Ditch	50	48.54	2.74	0.631	0.303
Vertical acetabular diameter	No lesion	54	50.42	2.52		
	Tongue	41	49.93	2.85	0.675	
	Ditch	50	50.52	2.77	0.983	0.582
Acetabular inclination angle	No lesion	54	68.50	4.95		
	Tongue	41	72.17	6.01	**0.006**	
	Ditch	50	72.19	4.49	**0.003**	1.000
Acetabular version angle	No lesion	54	44.72	4.89		
	Tongue	41	48.18	4.57	**0.001**	
	Ditch	50	48.49	3.89	**P<0.001**	0.948
Acetabular depth	No lesion	54	20.92	1.79		
	Tongue	41	20.91	2.07	1.000	
	Ditch	50	21.96	1.87	**0.023**	**0.036**

Table 4.4.4. Acetabular metrical and angular characteristics by FHNL, European American only.

Measurement	European American only				P Value	
	Lesions group	N	Mean	SD	No lesion	Tongue
Bi-acetabular depth distance	No lesion	56	151.93	8.72		
	Tongue	80	150.63	8.56	0.737	
	Ditch	59	153.77	11.29	0.584	0.160
Bi-acetabular rim distance	No lesion	56	187.49	10.16		
	Tongue	80	188.73	9.38	0.805	
	Ditch	59	190.86	12.98	0.248	0.516
Horizontal acetabular diameter	No lesion	56	50.96	4.61		
	Tongue	80	52.38	4.03	0.156	
	Ditch	59	53.06	4.02	**0.029**	0.639
Vertical acetabular diameter	No lesion	56	53.45	4.46		
	Tongue	80	53.88	3.89	0.837	
	Ditch	59	54.99	4.03	0.136	0.288
Acetabular inclination angle	No lesion	56	66.25	4.44		
	Tongue	80	67.11	5.49	0.677	
	Ditch	59	66.24	6.56	1.000	0.663
Acetabular version angle	No lesion	56	45.34	4.52		
	Tongue	80	46.73	4.50	0.211	
	Ditch	59	46.39	4.46	0.454	0.912
Acetabular depth	No lesion	56	22.04	2.43		
	Tongue	80	22.91	2.46	0.131	
	Ditch	59	23.46	2.41	**0.009**	**0.416**

Table 4.4.5. Acetabular metrical and angular characteristics by FHNL, African American only.

| Measurement | African American only | | | | P Value | |
	Lesions group	N	Mean	SD	No lesion	Tongue
Bi-acetabular depth distance	No lesion	58	144.72	7.76		
	Tongue	53	144.55	10	0.995	
	Ditch	61	145.26	9.42	0.950	0.919
Bi-acetabular rim distance	No lesion	58	178.81	8.45		
	Tongue	53	180.79	12.05	0.603	
	Ditch	61	180.10	10.30	0.793	0.940
Horizontal acetabular diameter	No lesion	58	51.01	3.74		
	Tongue	53	51.72	4.45	0.633	
	Ditch	61	50.32	3.48	0.628	0.164
Vertical acetabular diameter	No lesion	58	54.09	4.28		
	Tongue	53	54.10	7.23	1.000	
	Ditch	61	52.52	6.36	0.125	0.135
Acetabular inclination angle	No lesion	58	69.62	4.28		
	Tongue	53	67.75	7.23	0.272	
	Ditch	61	68.43	6.36	0.568	0.836
Acetabular version angle	No lesion	58	46.30	4.40		
	Tongue	53	46.93	4.94	0.772	
	Ditch	61	47.47	4.41	0.383	0.821
Acetabular depth	No lesion	58	22.08	1.83		
	Tongue	53	22.49	2.21	0.564	
	Ditch	61	22.99	2.03	0.053	0.429

Table 4.4.6. Acetabular metrical and angular characteristics by FHNL, European American males only.

| Measurement | European American males only | | | | P Value | |
	Lesions group	N	Mean	SD	No lesion	Tongue
Bi-acetabular depth distance	No lesion	30	150.50	8.71		
	Tongue	55	149.53	8.48	0.907	
	Ditch	42	152.90	11.66	0.588	0.242
Bi-acetabular rim distance	No lesion	30	189.59	9.54		
	Tongue	55	190.50	9.55	0.934	
	Ditch	42	191.94	13.02	0.664	0.811
Horizontal acetabular diameter	No lesion	30	53.78	3.59		
	Tongue	55	54.40	2.79	0.690	
	Ditch	42	54.61	3.35	0.553	0.951
Vertical acetabular diameter	No lesion	30	56.50	3.68		
	Tongue	55	55.63	3.03	0.542	
	Ditch	42	56.51	3.63	1.000	0.459
Acetabular inclination angle	No lesion	30	65.84	4.33		
	Tongue	55	65.35	5.06	0.910	
	Ditch	42	63.89	5.14	0.260	0.355
Acetabular version angle	No lesion	30	46.75	3.44		
	Tongue	55	46.30	4.43	0.900	
	Ditch	42	45.91	4.61	0.716	0.905
Acetabular depth	No lesion	30	23.27	2.22		
	Tongue	55	23.74	2.13	0.625	
	Ditch	42	24.20	2.13	0.200	0.590

Table 4.4.7. Acetabular metrical and angular characteristics by FHNL, African American males only.

| Measurement | African American males only | | | | P Value | |
	Lesions group	N	Mean	SD	No lesion	Tongue
Bi-acetabular depth distance	No lesion	30	141.53	6.78		
	Tongue	37	144.17	8.47	0.361	
	Ditch	28	142.91	6.73	0.782	0.799
Bi-acetabular rim distance	No lesion	30	179.01	8.25		
	Tongue	37	182.63	10.48	0.310	
	Ditch	28	181.34	9.57	0.652	0.865
Horizontal acetabular diameter	No lesion	30	53.54	2.99		
	Tongue	37	53.69	3.17	0.978	
	Ditch	28	52.83	2.54	0.661	0.511
Vertical acetabular diameter	No lesion	30	57.18	3.65		
	Tongue	37	55.96	2.80	0.262	
	Ditch	28	55.32	2.48	0.069	0.702
Acetabular inclination angle	No lesion	30	69.13	3.80		
	Tongue	37	65.04	5.04	**0.002**	
	Ditch	28	63.92	4.32	**P<0.001**	0.609
Acetabular version angle	No lesion	30	46.89	4.24		
	Tongue	37	46.06	4.88	0.746	
	Ditch	28	45.72	4.47	0.622	0.964
Acetabular depth	No lesion	30	22.91	1.53		
	Tongue	37	23.28	1.82	0.697	
	Ditch	28	24.02	1.91	0.063	0.252

Table 4.4.8. Acetabular metrical and angular characteristics by FHNL, European American females only.

| Measurement | European American females only | | | | P Value | |
	Lesions group	N	Mean	SD	No lesion	Tongue
Bi-acetabular depth distance	No lesion	26	153.58	8.60		
	Tongue	25	153.06	8.38	0.979	
	Ditch	17	155.94	10.35	0.703	0.599
Bi-acetabular rim distance	No lesion	26	185.06	10.50		
	Tongue	25	184.83	7.82	0.997	
	Ditch	17	188.21	12.87	0.619	0.581
Horizontal acetabular diameter	No lesion	26	47.70	3.34		
	Tongue	25	47.92	2.41	0.964	
	Ditch	17	49.23	2.84	0.247	0.362
Vertical acetabular diameter	No lesion	26	50.04	2.24		
	Tongue	25	50.01	2.58	0.999	
	Ditch	17	51.26	2.03	0.256	0.244
Acetabular inclination angle	No lesion	26	66.73	4.61		
	Tongue	25	70.98	4.36	**0.013**	
	Ditch	17	72.05	6.17	**0.004**	0.793
Acetabular version angle	No lesion	26	43.71	5.11		
	Tongue	25	47.66	4.58	**0.014**	
	Ditch	17	47.59	3.94	**0.034**	0.999
Acetabular depth	No lesion	26	20.63	1.85		
	Tongue	25	21.06	2.15	0.753	
	Ditch	17	21.04	2.14	0.288	0.664

Table 4.4.9. Acetabular metrical and angular characteristics by FHNL, African American females only.

| Measurement | African American females only | | | | P Value | |
	Lesions group	N	Mean	SD	No lesion	Tongue
Bi-acetabular depth distance	No lesion	28	148.15	7.36		
	Tongue	16	145.42	13.17	0.702	
	Ditch	33	147.25	10.92	0.945	0.845
Bi-acetabular rim distance	No lesion	28	178.60	8.80		
	Tongue	16	176.52	14.55	0.836	
	Ditch	33	179.05	10.93	0.987	0.756
Horizontal acetabular diameter	No lesion	28	48.30	2.29		
	Tongue	16	47.15	3.55	0.417	
	Ditch	33	48.19	2.66	0.988	0.470
Vertical acetabular diameter	No lesion	28	50.78	2.75		
	Tongue	16	50	3.33	0.580	
	Ditch	33	50.20	3.05	0.716	0.928
Acetabular inclination angle	No lesion	28	70.14	4.75		
	Tongue	16	74.03	7.74	0.098	
	Ditch	33	72.26	5.20	0.351	0.594
Acetabular version angle	No lesion	28	45.66	4.56		
	Tongue	16	48.99	4.58	0.051	
	Ditch	33	48.95	3.84	**0.014**	0.999
Acetabular depth	No lesion	28	21.19	1.73		
	Tongue	16	20.67	1.99	0.675	
	Ditch	33	22.12	1.72	0.136	**0.035**

4.5 Logistic regression

In the final stage of the analysis, we carried out logistic regression (forward stepwise) which include the demographic parameters (sex, age, ethnicity) as well as the metric variables measured on the femur (nine measurements), pelvis (eight measurements), acetabulum (five measurements) and the sacrum (one measurement) in order to identify the most associated with the tongue type (Table 4.5.1) and the ditch type (Table 4.5.2).

Table 4.5.1: the most associated variables with the tongue type.

Measurements	B	S.E.	Wald	df	Sig.	Exp(B)	95.0% C.I.for EXP(B)	
							Lower	Uppe
Femoral neck shaft angle	.097	.029	10.955	1	.001	1.102	1.040	1.16
Femoral torsion top	-.088	.023	14.111	1	.000	.916	.875	.959
Sacral inclination angle	.278	.072	14.711	1	.000	1.320	1.145	1.52
Acetabular depth	.408	.088	21.741	1	.000	1.504	1.267	1.78

Table 4.5.2: the most associated variables with the ditch type.

Measurements	B	S.E.	Wald	df	Sig.	Exp(B)	95.0% C.I.for EXP(B)	
							Lower	Uppe
Minimum femoral neck length	.163	.029	31.866	1	.000	1.177	1.112	1.24
Femoral neck shaft angle	.070	.029	6.008	1	.014	1.073	1.014	1.13
Vertical acetabular diameter	-.225	.054	17.520	1	.000	.799	.719	.887
Horizontal acetabular diameter	.067	.031	4.663	1	.031	1.070	1.006	1.13

4.6. Soft tissue and FHNL (cadaver study).

The hip joints of 12 cadavers were carefully dissected and analyzed for the presence of FHNL. The dissections revealed a close association between various anatomical structures and FHNL, as enumerated below.

4.6.1. Ditch type: This lesion was found to be associated with an extensive thickening of the deep layers of the circular fibers (zona orbicularis) surrounding the femoral neck (Figure 52).

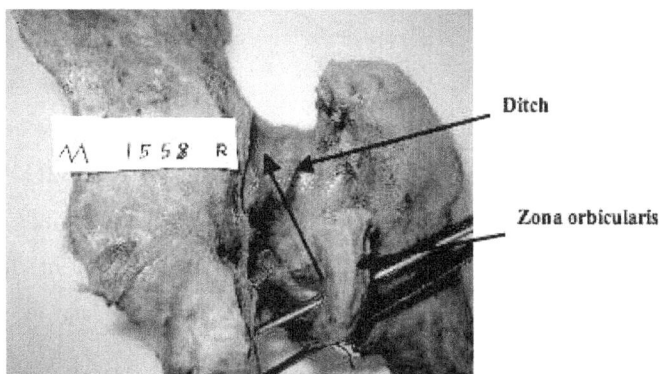

Figure 52: Thickening of the zona orbicularis (arrows) associated with the ditch type lesion (author work).

4.6.2. Tongue type: This lesion was associated with extensive friction between the femoral head-neck junction area and the acetabular rim (labrum) (Figure 53).

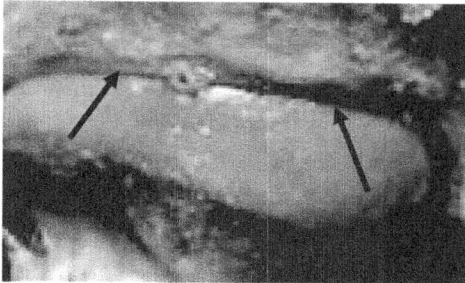

Figure 53: The acetabular labrum in contact with the femoral head (arrows) (author work).

4.6.3. Indentate type: The indentation is caused by pressure on the head of the femur from the iliopsoas tendon. The iliopsas tendon is located at the iliopsoas bursa, where the capsule of the hip joint, between the pubofemoral ligament and iliofemoral ligament, is thinnest (Figure 54 a and b).

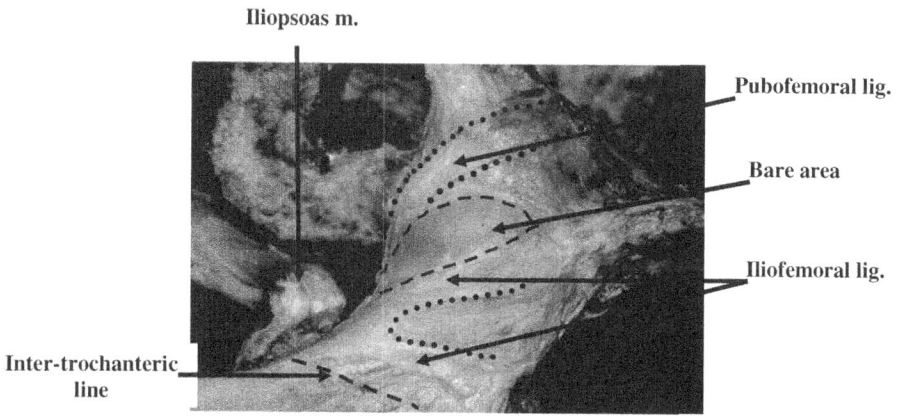

Figure 54 a: The tendon of the iliopsoas muscle crosses the bare area. The iliopsoas bursa is situated between the ligament of the muscle and the capsule (author work).

125

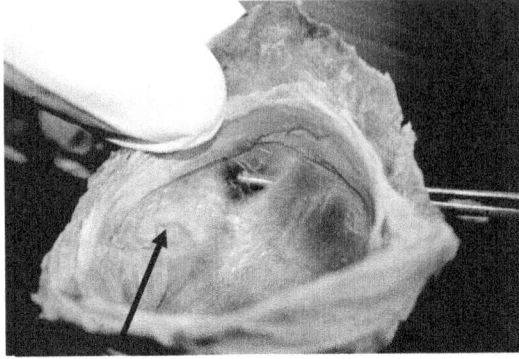

Figure 54 b: The hip joint capsule. Note how thin the capsule (bare area) is, behind the tendon of the iliopsoas muscle (arrow) (author work).

5. DISCUSSION

The current discussion focuses on two major issues: a- definitions for the various FHNLs and their demographic characteristics, and b- the possible etiology and pathophysiology of these lesions.

5.1 Demographical characteristic of FHNLs

Due to large variation in sample size, composition (sex ratio, age distribution) and geographical origin of the populations studied, prevalence of FHNLs varies largely among studies. Other factors that could have biased the numbers are the condition of the bones, namely whether they were fresh (with cartilage still intact) or dry (osteological collection), and how the researcher defined the lesion. For example, Odgers (1931) data is based on a study carried out on 52 femora only, all derived from the dissecting room. These implies fresh bone (soft tissue covering the underlying osseous changes) and aged biased sample (mainly elderly). The terminology used by Odgers (1931) referred to "eminentia" and "empreinte". Yet, "eminentia" and "poirier's facet are not the same entity: the eminentia refers to a strong bony ridge that runs from the anterior tubercle of the inter-trochanteric line to the head of the femur (and is seen in most individuals), while Poirier facet is simply an extension of the femoral head articular surface, overlapping part of the eminentia.

Considering the ambiguity in definitions of FHNLs, the differences in the demographic composition of the sample studied and the type of bone utilized (fresh or dry), the great inconsistency in the literature in regard to the prevalence of these phenomena is not surprising. Fick (1904) found 92% of bony facet (Poirier) in males femora. Parsons (1914) found the facet in 79% of males femora and in 58% of females right femur and 67% of females left femora. Parsons (1915) found a rate of 35.9% in males and 12% in females of Poirier facet in British Femora, and a much lower rate: 15.8% in males and 11.8% in females in historical Egyptian population femora. According to Pearson and Bell (1919) this facet is found in 87.8% of males and 79.9% of females in modern population.

In Odgers' population of cadavers, 35.9% of the male individuals manifested Poiriers' facet (tongue) and 10% of the females. No age effect was noted in regard to this trait. Allens' fossa was present in 92% of males and 67.5% of females. Odgers (1931) also noted that the older the individual, the deeper is the empriente (fossa). Additionally, the expression of the eminentia (facet) was found to be similar in the right and left side. Meyer (1934) found Poirier facet in 65.6% of his femora, and Allens' fossa in 26.8% right femur and 14.3% in the left femur.

Kostick (1963) found Poiriers' fact to be more common in the males compared with females (56% vs. 38% in Series A and 72% vs. 52% in Series I.D.H) and cervical imprint more common in females compared with males (45% vs. 29% in series A and 52% vs. 57% in Series I. D. H). His numbers in Table 2 (his original articles) do not support his conclusions.

Angel (1964) found the fossa of Allen to be very common among prehistoric Greeks, both in children (79%) and adult females (53%). The prevalence of this lesion decreases in frequency among male adults of later periods (Historic/Roman periods) – to ca. 13%. Plaque on the other hand, increased from 13% among prehistoric populations to 26% in the Roman period. In modern Americans, the fossa of Allen occurs in only about 10% (no differences between African American and European American). According to Angel, their severity is less marked compared to historical populations. Nevertheless, plaque show different behavior: 74% of modern male Americans, regardless of ethnicity, manifest a plaque whereas only 13% of prehistoric individuals and 27% individuals of the Roman period Greek populations manifest this trait. Plaque prevalence among ancient Greek female populations was very small (ca. 8%), whereas in modern American females the prevalence is relatively high: ranging from 55% to 63%. Angel attributed the differences between historic Greek and modern American populations to differences in life style and age structure (on the average, ancient Greeks lived 30 years less than modern Americans). As for Poiriers' facet, according to Angel this trait is found in similar frequencies in both historic Greek male populations (69-64%) and modern White Americans (69%), Black males present with somewhat higher incidence of Poirier facet (83%). Females manifest slightly smaller incidence of Poiriers'facet compared to males in both historic populations (64%-56%) and modern females Americans (56% in White females and 78% in Black females). According to Angel (1964), Poiriers' facet is less related to age or environment than is the reaction area. In our study, 72.9% of all individuals studied manifest some kind of a lesion on the femoral head-neck junction, the rate is higher for males (78%) compared to females (64.9%), and is in a general agreement with other studies. Similar to other studies, our "Tongue" (partially correspond to Poiriers' facet) is more common in males then females (37.3% vs. 24.3%), whereas the "Ditch" type (partially correspond to the fossa of Allen) is more common in females (33.7% vs. 26.7%). We also found that the "Ditch" (fossa) type occurs in similar percentages in Blacks and Whites males, but not the "Tongue" type: its prevalence is lower among male Blacks (32.4% vs. 41.2%). In females the situation is more complex as the "Tongue" type is more common in Whites (31.9% vs. 18%) while the "Ditch" type is more common in Blacks (39.6% vs. 26.4%). As we have shown, several previous studies suggest some association between FHNLs and age (e. g., Angel 1964), yet did not supply valid data to substantiate their claims. According to our data, "Tongue" prevalence increased from 24.2% in the 20-39 age cohort to 39.6% in the 60+ age cohort. "Ditch" prevalence on the other hand decreased with age, from 34.8% in the 20-39 age cohorts to 21.6% at the 60+ age group. This phenomenon is independent on sex and ethnicity. The "Tongue" type appears on both femora in 81.1% of the cases and the "Ditch" in 82.5%. Finnegan (1978) statistical analysis did not show neither side nor sex preference for fossa of Allen, Poiriers' facet and plaque. Correlation with age in his study was significant for the White sample only.

5.2. Etiology and pathophysiology of FHNL

Although the cervical fossa is commonly named after Allen who first mentioned the phenomenon (Allen, 1882), it was Bertraux (1891) who first suggested an explanation for this lesion, namely: due to the insertion of a strong fasciculus from the articular capsule. Poirier (1911) claimed that he could not find any evidence for "capsular fascicularis" at this region, a claim later on supported by Meyer (1934). Poirier (1911) himself suggested that the facet is formed due to a contact between the medial area of the femoral neck with the superior portion of the glenoidal lip in flexion of the thigh to a right angle. Fick (1904) has pointed out that considerable abduction combined with internal rotation would also be necessary before this contact could take place. Walmsley (1915) refuted this explanation, stating that "...in no natural position of any of the joints could this excursion (Poirier facet), in any of the specimens in which it was present, be made to enter the acetabular cavity" (p.310). He also excluded the possibility that the iliopsoas muscle was responsible for this facet, and suggested that the vertical limb of the ilio-femoral ligament in the position of complete extension is involved in creating this facet. Walmsley (1915) maintained that the vertical limb of the ilio-femoral ligament, in the position of complete extension, is responsible for the "empriente". This explanation was criticized by Meyer (1924) on the ground that: a- there is no other place in the body where a pressure from a moving ligament produces a roughening of the underlying bony surface; b- why is the lateral part of the eminence smooth, while only the inner part is eroded, if capsular pressure is responsible for both?; c-the main direction of the "empriente" usually makes an angle with this limb of Bigelow's ligament. Meyer in a later article (1934) also rejected Poirier hypothesis on the ground that no anatomical connection between these two anatomical structures occurs under this condition (except when someone is lying on the side).

Odgers (1931) divided the causes for "empreinte" into two major categories. In the first category he included the study of Poirier (1911), Tramond and Evangeli (1894) and Regnault (1901) that suggested that this lesion resulted from the rubbing of the acetabular margin against the upper part of the femoral neck (mainly in exaggerated flexion of the thigh on the pelvis). In the second category he included the studies of Fick (1904), Parsons (1916) and Walmsley (1915) who claimed that medial rotation with extreme flexion are necessary to get the facet and acetabular border into contact. According to Odgers (1931), the condition described in the second model is more appropriate, nevertheless this "is obviously a most unnatural position for any person to adopt" (p. 360). It is important to note that Pearson (1919) and Meyer (1924) claimed that such contact may occur during sleep (lying full length on the side in bed with the upper lower limb thrown forward) and, therefore, there is no need to find a habitual posture likely to produce Poirier's facet. Odgers (1931) dismissed the first explanation by claiming that the fibro-cartilaginous acetabular rim is not capable of making marked erosion as often seen, and therefore some kind of movement must be involved. The second category according to Odgers (1931) related the cause of "empriente" to friction between the iliopsoas tendon and the anterior part of the capsule of the hip (over the femoral neck). Odgers (1931) rejected this hypothesis on the ground that the tendon of the iliopsoas is medial to the "empriente" and, when the "bursa beneath the tendon communicate with the joint, it is the lateral part of the head of the bone which is exposed. Odgers (1931) also rejected earlier claims made by Meyer (1924) that the hip joint presents a unique situation of such friction,so unique that it occurs only one other place in the body, that being between the head of the astragalus and the spring ligament where erosion of the cartilage was also noted. In his explanation for FHNLs, Odgers followed Parsons (1915) study who showed that the ridge on the front of the neck (correspond to Walmsley's capsular ridge) is the outer limit of the groove transmitting the band of the zonular fibers which embrace the head of the femur lateral to the articular area. At the upper border of the neck, this stout band (zona orbicularis) broadens and comes in close contact with the neck. Odgers (1931) claimed that in all his cadavers the band indeed laid in cervical erosion. Odgers (1931) summarized his observation by stating that both the face (Poirier) and the erosion "empriente" were due to the same agent. The fibro-cartilage extension, according to Odgers develops as a protection against the friction, and the erosion is the breakdown of this protection (Meyers basic argument was that capsular friction cannot make one part smooth and another part rough). The reason for the different prevalence of "empriente" between the genders is due, according to Odgers (1931) to the different amount of pressure applied to this area by the capsule. The degree of the osseous changes at this region according to Odgers depends on two factors: The thickening of the zona orbicularis and the thickness of the "eminentia" (ignoring the fact that facets may also appear on the posterior aspect of the neck where the "eminentia" is usually absent).

Odgers wrote: "the essential factor in the production of any secondary groove or ridge on a bone must, surely, be movement", and this happens by a momentary contact between the femoral neck and the zona at the end of the step in walking. Meyer (1934) forcefully objected to this approach stating that "I have never seen the slightest evidence that such a depression as a fossa of Allen or the deeper and larger 'excavation,' could be produced by erosion from friction" (p. 488). Furthermore, the zona orbicularis, according to Meyer is thicker posteriorly while Allens' fossa is located anteriorly, and that "A deep fossa often is present when the zona is grossly absent" (p. 497). He also claimed that the zona fibers are thicker internally, causing friction, and that the presence of a cervical ridge cannot be explained by the zona friction. What Meyer basically stated is that Allens' fossa could not have been excavated by the zona (which is much softer than the underlying bone) but is due to absorption – in consequence of pressure atrophy "due to some other cause" (p. 503). This pressure is not due to increasing tension of capsule in walking but sustained pressure "such as that from the glenoid lip in connection with relatively long-maintained postures such as lying on the side" (p. 503). In response to Odgers (1931), he continued by saying that in his 1924 paper he did not suggest that the fossa is being produced during sleep..."I suggested that they resulted from absorption due to pressure" ..."and that such soft structure as the joint capsule could not possibly erode a fibro-cartilage' and the far more resistant underlying bone, as Odgers implies" (p.488). Meyer (1934) claimed that some of the impressions seen on the neck of the femur are not due to erosion or atrophy, but mainly to molding during growth. Poirier facet, according to Meyer, is a molding process resulting from the contact between the ligamentous acetabular lip and the femoral neck. He strengthened his argument by stating that if it was due to the friction of the zona orbicularis, the direction of this elevated bony ramp was antero-posteriorly (parallel to direction of the zona fibers) and not medio-lateral. Meyer (1934) claimed that although Poirier facet and Allen fossa occur in the same place on the femoral neck, they do not occur at the same time.

He suggested that the same agent is responsible for both phenomenon, yet evoking different reaction (due to different intensity and duration during different periods of life). Meyer (1934) also claim that the term 'empreiente' (impression) used by both Poirier and Bertaux is misleading, as sometime the area is elevated ('bourrelet').

The notion that the fossa is producing when lying on the side was first suggested by Pearson and Bell (1919), and rediscovered by Meyer in 1924. Odgers (1931) attacked Meyer for not mentioning that this hypothesis is not his. Meyer (1934) in a later reply claimed that although Pearson and Bell indeed presented this theory, at the end of their paper they dismissed it. Meyer summarized his conclusions as follows: "...the cervical ridge and the raised facets in this region of the neck of the femur, may be due to bone formation by the irritated periosteum and that the fossa of Allen and, partly, also the deeper and longer incisions may have resulted from bone resorption from pressure of the acetabular lip in the lying posture with the extremity flexed." (p. 506)...."It is the contact of the ligamentous acetabular lip with the neck of the femur that is the chief factor in the prevention of forward rotation when lying on the side during sleep..." (p. 507). Kostick (1963) attributed Poiriers' facet to the rubbing of the cervical eminence against the capsule in hip extension (especially the iliofemoral ligament). He also refuted the hypothesis that the squatting position can contribute to the development of Poirier facet.

Angel (1964) claimed that Poirier (1911), Meyer (1924) and Fick (1904) explanation for the formation of Poiriers' facet (extreme flexion plus internal rotation) should be rejected as "no human being even in childhood sleeps with his thighs tight against his chest" (p. 131). He further claimed that the iliopsoas tendon crosses the hip joint too far medially to have a causal effect on the reaction area. Angel (1964) also dismissed Sudeck (1899) hypothesis that the reaction area marks the line of last ossification. Angel (1964) adopted Odgers (1931) approach and suggested that the direct causal agent is the hip joint capsule, mainly the zona orbicularis (which tighten around the neck in full extension). Angel who differentiates between Poiriers' facet and what he called "reaction area" suggesting that Poiriers' facet is created when the femoral head-neck junction rubs against the acetabulum, the labrum and probably the iliopsoas tendon, whereas the reaction area (plaque and fossa) is in contact only with the capsule of the hip joint. Angel hypothesized that the friction process (between the zona and the neck) produces first a local atrophy (Fossa of Allen) and then in the middle age a hypertrophic response (plaque) at the reaction area.. What cause this reaction area? No muscles or tendons are attached to this area and contact of the reaction area with the acetabulum or acetabular labrum can occur only in extreme positions of flexion and internal rotation. Is the explanation proposed by Angel (1964) is satisfactory? Was Walmsley (1915) right in suggesting that the surface reaction results from mechanical, abrasive effect of adjacent overlying hip capsule, which is particularly thick in this region due to crossing of circular and vertical fibers (zona orbicularis) and lateral part of the ilio-femoral ligament with additional indirect pressure applied by the overlying straight head of the rectus femoris muscle and by the more laterally positioned iliopsoas muscle? Is Walmsley hypothesis regarding an association between the prominence of the reaction area and the thickness and roughness of the underlying capsule substantial?

5.3. FHNLs and femur and pelvic morphometrics

Angel failed to show morphometrical differences in the femur between those who manifest a reaction area and those who did not. He concluded that "the development of the reaction area is not a result of special body structure or of static posture and must be a result of dynamic factors primarily in the interaction of muscles (iliopsoas) and ligaments (zona) with gravity and leverage in extreme extension and secondary in arrangement of ligament fibers in the capsule (crossing of the zona and the iliofemoral ligament)." (p. 139). Modern medical/radiological studies suggested some association between the femur architecture and the development of femoral acetabular impingement (FAI), but fail to supply solid data to support such claim. Our detailed study of more than 400 femora has revealed the followings: Individuals with tongue or ditch lesions have significantly longer femurs (anatomical and physiological length) and longer necks compared with individuals with no lesion, no significant differences in these two parameters were found between the tongue and

134

the ditch group. On the other hand, femoral neck shaft angle was significantly greater in the ditch type group compared to the tongue and no lesion group. This data suggest an involvement of biomechanical factors in the formation of FHNLs: the longer the femur, the greater the lever arm, henceforth the greater the stress on the femoral neck. The greater the femoral neck-shaft angle the greater the tension of the zona.

The biomechanical rational for the ditch lesion can be described as follows: it is not surprising that the ditch type is associated with valgus deformity (increase neck shaft angle) of the hip. In increase neck-shaft angle the femoral head is directed more superiorly in the acetabulum, resulting in many biomechanical attentions (Maquet, 1999; Pauwels, 1976). This alignment subjects the femoral neck to more compressive forces, and not less important it displaces the joint reaction force laterally in the acetabulum and is applied over a small joint surface, leading to increased joint stress (Oatis, 2009). Most of this stress is handled by the zona orbicularis, the outcome of which is constant friction between tighten zona and neck of femur.

In the same token, the tongue, type can be explained as follows:

The lengthing neck in the tongue type implies that the trochanter in further away from the joint centers, affectively lengthening the moment arm of the hip abductors. Although this puts the hip abductors at a mechanical advantage, it also tends to increase the medial pull of the femur into the acetabulum, leadings to a forced contact between the acetabular osteological rim and labrum and the femoral neck (Maquet, 1999) Not surprisingly this lesion is associated with acetabular orientation and depth.

Additionally, size and shape of the pelvis was not associated with FHNLs. The only parameter that shows a relationship to FHNLs was sacral inclination which was significantly greater in the ditch group. This also attests to a greater stress on the zona orbicularis in individuals with Ditch. The two metric parameters of the acetabulum that were found to be associated with FHNLs (ditch and tongue) were acetabular depth and acetabular inclination angle. This is not surprising as both traits facilitate a contact between the acetabular rim and femoral head-neck area. These findings are in concordance with some previous medical studies that suggested that acetabular structure and position may play a role in FAI. It seems that acetabular version angle also plays a role in FHNLs formation, but the data is not conclusive.

5.4 Pathophysiology of FHNLs – summary

Following the results of our dissections and morphometrical analysis, we propose explanations for the various FHNLs phenomena (Figure 55).

The ditch lesion is strongly associated with certain morphological traits of the femur and the acetabulum (e.g., femoral length, neck-shaft angle, acetabular inclination). The combination of these traits exposes the upper-anterior section of the femoral capsule, mainly the zona orbicularis, to excessive tension. With time, the continued strong friction between the zona and the neck create a deep ditch at the femoral head-neck junction (Figure 56). The tongue lesion is due to continued contact between the acetabular labrum and the femoral neck. What contributes most to this contact is the inclination of the acetabulum (Figure 57). The sunken lesion is independent of the pelvis, femur or acetabular size and shape. It is created by retinacular fibers that transmit blood to the femoral head (Figure 58). The indentate lesion is due to a strong pressure applied by the iliopsoas muscle (tendon) on the femoral head (Figure 59).

Combining all the evidence available, it is clear that the femoral lesions described in this study are not in earlier expression of some hip joint diseases, but rather the diseases themselves.

Odgers' Model

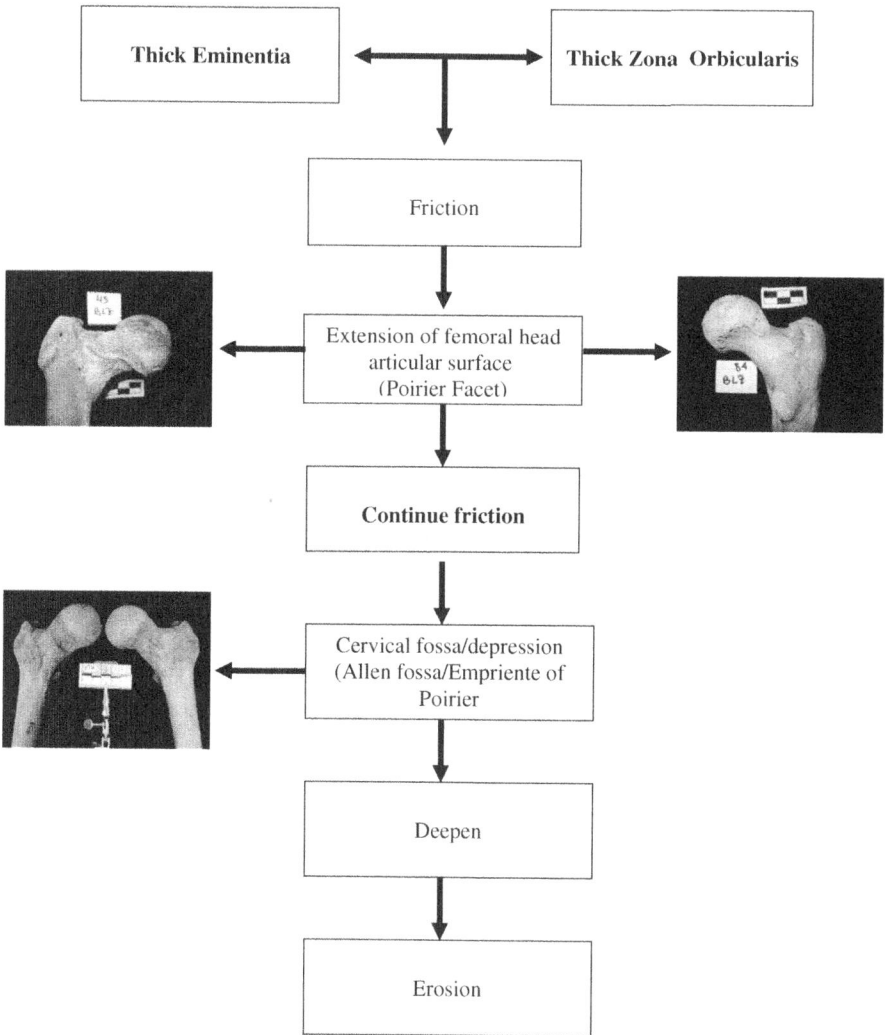

Figure 55: The processes by which Poiriers fact and Allens fossa are formed, according to Odgers 1931.

The Ditch model

Pelvis size and shape	Acetabular size and shape	Femoral size and shape	External muscles and ligaments

Sacral inclination angle	1. Acetabular inclination 2. Acetabular version 3. Acetabular depth	1. Femoral neck length (M) 2. Femoral anat. Length 3. Femoral neck-shaft angle	Thickening of zona orbicularis

Increase contact between zona and head-neck junction	Increase lever arm Strong friction between zona and neck

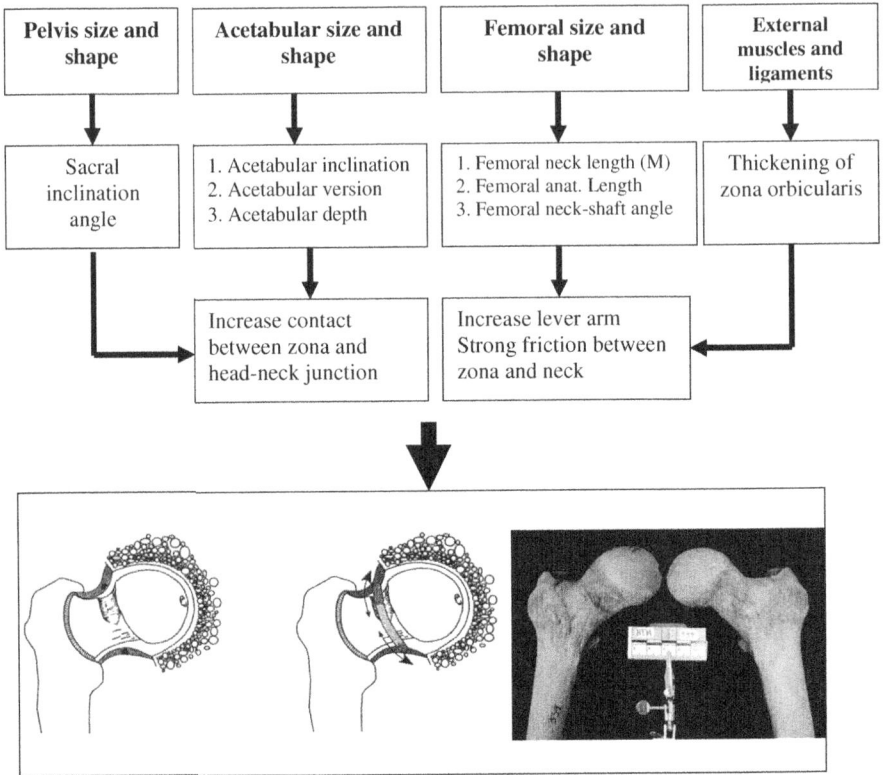

Figure 56: A model describing the development of the 'Ditch' type lesions, based on morphometrical and anatomical studies carried out in this research.

The tongue model

Pelvis size and shape	Acetabular size and shape	Femoral size and shape	External muscles and ligaments
No effect	1. Acetabular inclination 2. Acetabular version (F)	Femoral neck length	Labrum
	Linear contact between acetabular rim and head-neck junction	Increase lever arm Strong friction between labrum and neck	

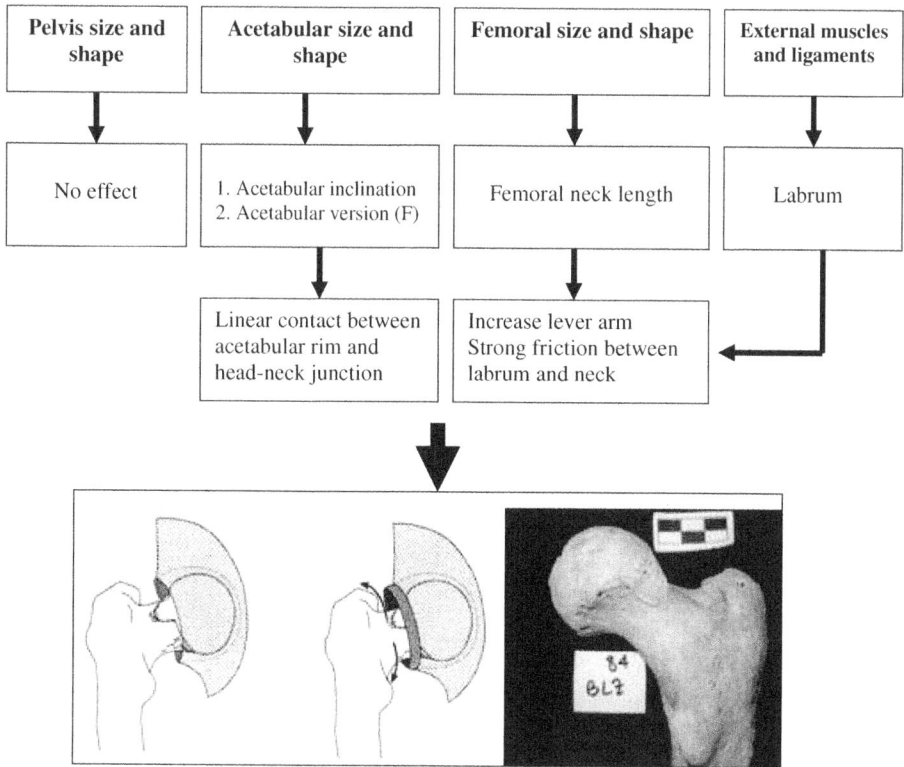

Figure 57: A model describing the development of the 'Tongue' type lesions, based on morphometrical and anatomical studies carried out in this research.

The Sunken model

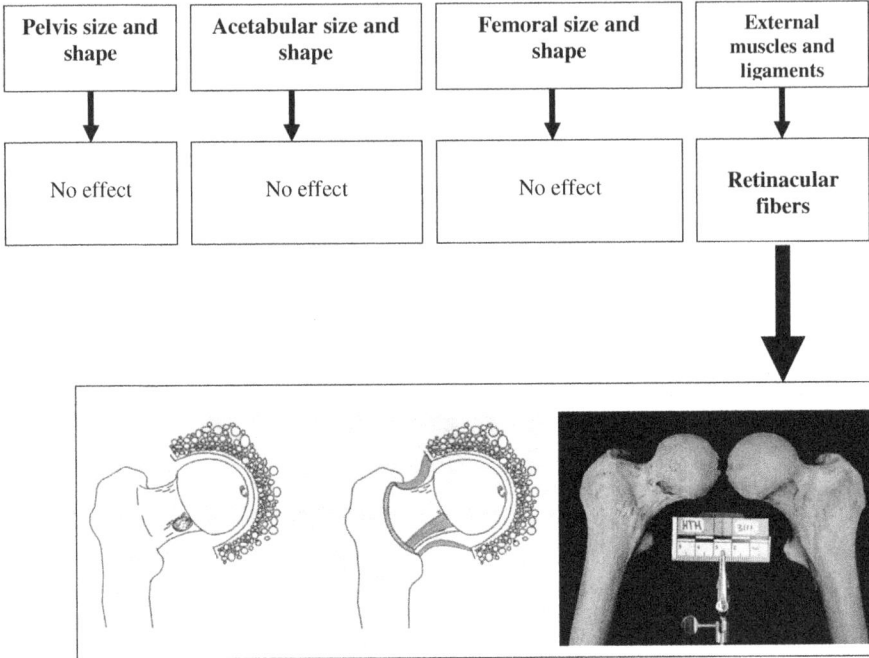

Figure 58: A model describing the development of the 'Sunken' type lesions, based on morphometrical and anatomical studies carried out in this research.

The indentate model

Pelvis size and shape	Acetabular size and shape	Femoral size and shape	External muscles and ligaments
↓	↓	↓	↓
No effect	No effect	No effect	Iliopsoas muscle

Increase lever arm
Strong friction between iliopsoas tendon and femoral head

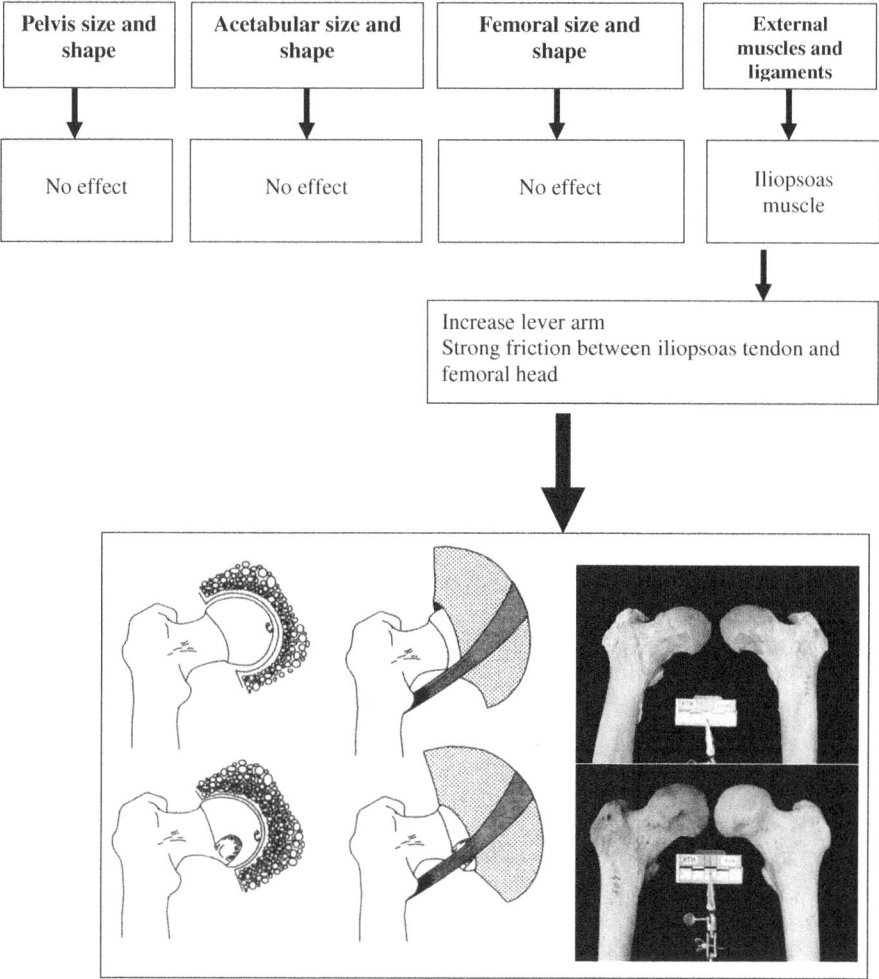

Figure 59: A model describing the development of the 'Indentate' type lesions, based on morphometrical and anatomical studies carried out in this research.

5.5 Modern Medicine and FHNLs

As we have already mentioned in our introductory chapter, FHNL did not receive much attention from the medical community. The first serious effort was been made by Pitt et al. (1982) who examined A-P radiographs of adult femoral necks and identified a small well delineated rounded pit with sclerotic margin beneath the anterior cortex. The pit is formed by herniation of soft tissues (probably synovial tissue) through erosions or perforation of the reaction area surface, "which results from abrasive action of the overlying hip capsule" (p. 1116). The lesions were termed "herniation pit" and have been considered to be an incidental finding in 5% of the population of healthy individuals (Pitt et al., 1982). Other studies reported on a much higher prevalence (12%) of herniation pits (Daenen et al., 1997). Crabbe et al. (1992) claimed that this pit, unlike what was commonly believed, is not stable but rather can grow very rapidly. Although Pitt et al. (1982) and Daenen et al. (1997) studies did not indicate an underlying morphological disorder to these cystic lesions, they recognized that femoral alterations at the anterosuperior head-neck junction were present in most of these skeletons and that these changes are in the shape of "plaque" and "fossa". Two distinct type of FAI have been identified in the medical literature: **Femoral FAI** – caused by an abnormally shaped femoral head that has a peripherally increased radius thus causing acetabular rim damage as it enters the acetabulum during motion, especially flexion with internal rotation (Ito et al., 2001), **Acetabular FAI** – result of a linear contact between the acetabular rim and the femoral head-neck junction (cause: acetabular abnormality such as deep acetabular socket or acetabular retroversion). According to Ganz et al., (2003), in most cases of FAI, combined femoral and acetabular abnormalities can be found. Leunig et al. (2005) concluded that "on the basis of the radiographically depicted location of the fibrocystic alterations at the anterosuperior femoral neck and the reported location of herniation pits, it is very likely that herniation pits and FAI-induced fibrocysts are the same entity" (p. 244). Yet, the later believed that the pits are not due to synovial invagination but rather due to intraosseous ganglia.

It soon became a common notion that FAI occurs when there is a conflict between the proximal femur and the acetabular rim (Ganz et al., 2003), and that FAI is a cause of premature osteoarthritis of the hip (Wagner et al., 2003). Today, FAI is divided to two categories based on the dominate structure involved: **cam FAI** – is due to nonspherical shape of the femoral head and reduced depth of the femoral waist which lead to abutment of the femoral head-neck junction against the acetabular rim (Ito et al., 2001), **pincer FAI** – where acetabular overcoverage limits the range of motion and leads to a conflict between the acetabulum and the femur (Gantz et al., 2003), usually associated with deep acetabulum and posteroinferior acetabular cartilage lesions (Pfirrmann et al., 2006). The identification of FAI is important clinically as it dictate the type of surgery applied (Pfirrmann et al., 2006).

Ito et al. (2001) found that patients with cam FAI manifest a significant reduction in mean depth of the femoral waist at the anterior aspect of the femoral neck when compared with that in patients with pincer FAI. Based on Giori and Trousdale (2003) study, this can contribute to overcoverage of the acetabulum and hence to pincer FAI (and hence to osteoarthritis). Other factors that may be involved are labral tears (Wenger et al. (2004), ossification of the acetabular rim, os acetabuli (Kassarjian et al., 2005) and bump deformity (Jager et al., 2004).

In 1975 Stuhlberg et al described the femoral head-neck bump deformity as a "pistol-grip deformity" and reported its presence in 40% of all patients who developed osteoarthritis of the hip. With increasing interest in OA of the hip, attention has been paid also to other FHNLs. It was found that patients with OA in the hips suffer from femoroacetabular impingement (FAI), especially young individuals with nonspherical femoral head. It was noted that people with nonspherical femoral heads had a decreased head-neck offset, and that in these individuals the femoral head and neck will be forced against the acetabulum during flexion and internal rotation, known as the "cam-type impingement" mechanism (Ito et al., 2001). Siebenrock et al. (2004) claimed that in the majority of patients with nonspherical morphologic features of the head, the impinging anterosuperior portion of the femoral head corresponds to a triangular-shaped extension of the femoral head cartilage onto the neck (meaning

Poirier facet). The authors suggested that growth abnormality of the capital physis as one probable underlying cause for a nonspherical head. Leunig et al., 2005 reported an association between fibrocystic changes at the anterosuperior femoral neck and femoroacetabular impingement. In recent years some orthopedic surgeons adopted an operative treatment to reduce femoroacetabulr impingement (Jager et al., 2004). It is generally believe that femoroacetabular impingement is often associated with reduced femoral anteversion or an osseous bump on the femoral head-neck junction. Impingement symptoms can be caused by a variety of causes: chronic slipped capital femoral epiphysis, reduced antetorsion of the femoral neck, protrusion acetabuli, elliptical femoral head, and decreased anterior femoral offset.

Ito et al (2009) were the first to experiment on the role of the zona orbicularis, the labrum and the capsular ligamentous complexes (mainly iliofemoral and ischiofemoral) in hip joint stability. They found that the proximal to middle part of the capsule, which includes the zona orbicularis, was the most important structure for hip stability.

6. Main findings of the study.

The current study revealed six major findings in regard to FHNL: a- the phenomenon is much more common than previously appreciated; b- there are more types (six) of FHN lesions than previously reported, and these types vary largely in prevalence; c- some of the FHN lesions are sex, age and ethnicity dependent; d- Archaeological populations manifest different pattern of FHNL compared to modern populations; e- there is clear association between the architecture of the femur and the acetabulum and the type of lesion; f- each lesion is caused by a different mechanism that involve forced contact between adjacent anatomical structures.

References

Adna S, Svenningsen S, Dale LG, Benum P. 1986. The acetabular sector angle of the adult hip determined by computed tomography. Acta Radiol Diagn .p: 443-447.

Aiello L, Dean C. 1990. Human Evolution Anatomy. The hominoid femur. Academic Press Limited p: 436-438.

Allen H. 1882. A system of human anatomy. Sec. II. Bones and joints. Philadelphia.

Angel JL. 1964. The reaction area of the femoral neck. Clin Orthop 32:130-142.

Bergmann G, Deuretzbacher G, Heller M, Graichen F, Rohlmann A, Strauss J, Duda G.N. 2001. Hip contact forces and gait patterns from routine activities. J Biomechanics 34: 859-871.

Berry A, Berry R. 1967. Epigenetic variation in the human cranium. J Anat 101: 361-379.

Berry A, Berry R. 1971. Origins and relationships of the ancient Egyptians. In the population biology of ancient Egypt (ed. D. R. Brothwell and B. Chiarelli), pp. 199-208. London and New York: Academic press.

Bertaux T. 1891. Doctorate thesis in medicine. Lille

Bombelli R, Santore RF, Poss R. 1984. Mechanics of the normal and osteoarthritic hip. A new perspective. Clin Orthop.182:69-78.

Clark JM, Haynor DR. 1987. Anatomy of the abductor muscles of the hip as studied by computed tomography. J Bone Joint Surg 69: 1021-1031.

Crabbe JB, Martel W, Matthews LS. 1992. Rapid growth of femoral herniation pit. Am J Roentgenol. 159:1038-1040.

Cruvellhier J. 1862. Traite' Anatomie. descriptive, I, pp. 229-232.

Daenen B, Preidler KW, Padmanabhan S, Brossmann J, Tyson R, Goodwin DW, Bergman G, Resnick D. 1997. Symptomatic herniation pits of the femoral neck: anatomic and clinical stody. AJR Am J Roentgonol. 168:149-153.

Fick R. 1904. Handbuch der Anatomie und Mechanik der Gelenke 1: Teil: Anatomie der Gelenke. In: von Bardeleben K, ed Handbuch der Anatomie des Menschen. Jena: Gustav Fischer Verlag; 312-319.

Finnegan M. 1978. Non-metric variation of the infracranial skeleton. J Anat 125: 23-37.

Frankel VH. 1960. In the femoral neck: Function, Fracture mechanisms, Internal fixation. Springfield: Charles C. Thomas.

Fuss F, Bacher A. 1991. New aspects of the morphology and function of the human hip joint ligaments. Am J Anat 192:1-13.

Ganz R, Parvizi J, Beck M, Leunig M, Notzli H, Siebenrock K. 2003. Femoroacetabular impingement: a cause for osteoarthritis of the hip. Clin Orthop Relat Res. 417: 112-120.

Gardner E. 1948. The innervations of the hip-joint. Anat. Rec. p101:353.

Giori N, Trousdale R. 2003. Acetabular retroversion is associated with osteoarthritis of the hip. Clin Orthop Relat Res 417 : 263-269.

Gray H. 1985. Anatomy of the Human Body. 30th American Edition, Lea & FEBIGER, Philadelphia.

Henke W. 1863. Handbuch der Anatomie u. Mechanik der Gelenke, S. 279.

Henle J. 1871. Handbuch der systematischen Anatomie des Menschen. S.279.

Hewitt J, Guilak F, Glisson R, Vail TP. 2001. Regional material properties of the human hip joint capsule ligaments. Orthop Res J. 19: 359-364.

Howells W and Hotelling H. 1936. Mesurement and correlations on pelvis of Indians of southwest. Am J Phys Anthrop. 21: 91-106.

Ito K, Minka II MA, Leunig M, Ganz R. 2001. Femoroacetabular impingement and the cam-effect. J Bone Joint Surg. 83B: 171-176.

Ito H, Song Y, Lindsey D, Safran M, Giori N. 2009. The proximal hip joint and the zona orbicularis contribute to hip joint stability in distraction. J Orthop Res. Epub ahead of print.

Jager M, Wild A, Westhoff B, Krauspe R. 2004. Femoroacetabular impingement caused by a femoral osseous head-neck bump deformity: clinical, radiological, and experimental results. J Orthop Sci. 9: 256-263.

John H, Richard G, Farshid G, Parker TV. 2002. The mechanical properties of the human hip capsule ligaments. J Arthroplasty 17: 82-89.

Kapandji I. 1987. The physiology of the joints. Williams and Wilkins, Baltimore, vol. 2, 5th ed.

Kassarjian A, Yoon L, Belzile E, Connolly S, Millis M, Palmer W. 2005. Triad of MR arthrographic findings in patients with cam-type femoroacetabular impingement. Rdiology 236: 588-592.

Kempson GE, Spivey CJ, Swanson SA, Freeman MA. 1971. Patterns of cartilage stiffness on normal and degenerate human femoral heads. J Biomech 4: 597-609.

Kim YT, Azuma H. 1995. The nerve endings of the acetabular labrum. Clin Orthp 320: 176-181.

Kostick EL. 1963. Acets and imprints on the upper and lower extremities of femora from a western Nigerian population. J Anat 97:393-402.

Legaye J, Duval-Beaupere G, Hecquet G, Mrty C. 1998. Pelvic incidence: a fundamental pelvic parameter for three-dimensional regulation of spinal sagittal curves. Eur Spine J 7: 99-103.

Leunig M, Beck M, Woo A, Dora C, Kerboull M, Ganz R. 2003. Acetabular rim degeneration. Clin Orthop Relat Res. 413: 201-207.

Leunig M, Beck M, Kalhor M, Kim YJ, Werlen S, Ganz R. 2005. Fibrocystic changes at anterosuperior femoral neck: prevalence in hips with femoroacetabular impingement. Radiol 236: 237-246.

Levangie PK, Norkin CC. 2001. Joint Structure and Function. Philadelphia: F. A. Davis Company.

Lewinnek GE, Kelsey J, White AA, Kreiger NJ. 1980. The significance and a comparative analysis of the epidemiology of the hip fractures. Clin Orthop 152: 35-43.

Maquet P. 1999. Biomechanics of hip dysplasia. Acta Orthop Belg 65:302-314.

Masaaki M, Judy RF, William NC, James AD. 2001. Morphologic features of the acetabulum and femur. Clin Orthop Related Research 393: 52-65.

Masharawe Y, Peleg S, Hanne B, Dar G, Steingberg N, Medlej B, Abbas J, Salame K, Mirovski Y, Peled N, Hershkovitz I.2008. Facet asymmetry in normal vertebral growth: characterization and etiologic of scoliosis. Spine. 33: 898-902.

Mays S. 2006. Spondylolysis, spondylolisthesiss, and lubo-sacral morphology in medieval skeletal population. Am J Phys Antropol 131: 352-362.

McLaren RH. 1973. Prosthetic hip angulation. Radiol 107:705-706.

Meyer A. 1924. The "cervical fossa" of Allen. Am J Phys Anthrop. 7: 257-269

Meyer A. 1934. The genesis of the fossa of Allen and associated structures. Amer J Anat. 55: 469-510.

Moore K, Dally AL. 1999. Clinically Oriented Anatomy, 4th ed, Lippincott Williams & Wilkins: Philadelphia.

Oatis C. 2009. Kinosiology: the mechanics and pathomechanics of human movement, Second edition, Lippincott Williams & Wilkins, pp: 687-702.

Odgers PNB. 1931. Tow details about the neck of the femur: 1) the eminentia. 2) The empreinte. J Anat 65: 352-362.

Parsons F. 1914. The characters of the English thigh bone. J Anat Physiol 48: 238-267.

Parsons F. 1915. The characters of the English thigh bone. J Anat Physiol 4: 345-361.

Parsons F. 1916. The characters of the English thigh bone. Anat Soc. Vol. L. P.11.

Pauwels F. 1976. Biomechanics of the normal and diseased hip: theoretical foundation technique and resuls of treatment. An Atlas. Belin: Springer- Verlag, pp: 30-37.

Pearson K, Bell J. 1919. A study of the English thigh bone. J Anat Lond 48:238-267.

Peleg S, Dar G, Medlej B, Steinberg N, Masharawi Y, Latimer B, Jellema L, Peled N, Arensburg B, Hershkovitz I. 2007. Orientation of the human sacrum: Antropological perspectives and methodological approaches. Am J Phys Antropol 133: 967-977.

Pfirrmann C, Mengiardi B, Dora C, Kalberer F, Zanetti M, Hodler J. 2006. Cam and pincer Femoroacetabular impingement: characteristic MR arthrographic findings in 50 pationts.Radiology. 240: 778-785.

Pitt M, Graham A, Shipman J, Birkby W. 1982. Herniation pit of the femoral neck. Am J Roentgenol 138:1115-1121.

Poirier P. 1911. Traite′ d′anatomie Humaine (Poirier and Charpy), vol. I. Paris et Cie.

Radin E. 1979. Practical Biomechanics for the Orthopedic Surgeon. John Wiley & Sons, New York.

Regnault F. 1901. Bull.et mem de la Soc. d Anthropologie de Paris, 5th Series, Vol. XI p. 377.

Ruff C. 1995. Biomechanics of the hip and birth in early homo. Am J Phys Anthropol 98: 527-574.

Rushfeld PD, Mann, RW, Harris WH. 1979. Influence of cartilage geometry on the pressure distribution in the human hip joint. Science 204 (4391): 413-415.

Saudek C. 1985. The hip. In J. Gould, G.J. Davies (Eds). Orthopedic and Sports Physical Therapy. St. Louis: Mosby pp:365-407.

Schultz A. 1969. Observations on the acetabulum of primates. Folia Primatolo 11:181-199.

Siebenrock K, Schoeniger R, Ganz R. 2003. Anterior femoro-acetabular impingement due to acetabular retroversion. J Bone Surg Am 85-A(2): 278-86.

Siebenrock K, Wahab K, Werlen S, Kalhor M, Leuing M, Ganz R. 2004. Abnormal extension of the femoral head epiphysis as a cause of cam impingement. Clin Orthop Relat Res 418: 54-60.

Singleton HC, Leveau BF. 1975. The hip joint: structure, Stability and stress. Phys Ther 55: 957-973.

Soderberg G. 1986. Kinesiology: Application to Pathological Motion. Baltimore: Williams & Wilkins 21: 24-38.

Sudeck P. 1899. Zur Anatomie und aetiologie der coxa vara adolescentium zugleich ein beitrag zu der lehre von dem architektonischen Bau des coxalen femurendes, Arch. Clin Chirurg 59: 504.

Tague R. G. 1992. Sexual dimorphism in the human bony pelvis with a consideration of the Neandertal pelvis from Kebara cave, Israel. Am J Phys Anthrop. 88: 1-21.

Tan C, Wong WC. 1990. Absence of the ligament of the head of the femur in the human hip joint. Singapore Med J 31: 360-363.

Tayton E. 2007. Femoral anteversion: a necessary angle or an evolutionary vestige. J Bone Joint Surg 89: 1283-1288.

Thomason B, Silverman D, Walter D, Olshaker R. 1983. Focal bone tracer uptake associated with a herniation pit of the femoral neck. Clin Nucl Med 8: 304-305.

Tramond A and Evangeli. 1894. These pour le Doctorat en Medecine. Paris.

Wagner S, Hofstetter W, Chiquet M, Mainil-Varlet P, Stauffer E, Ganz R. 2003. Early osteoarthritic changes iof human femoral head cartilage supsequent to femoro-acetabular impingement Osteoarthritis Cartilage 11: 508-518.

Walmsley T. 1915. Observations on certain structural details of the neck of the femur. J Anat Lond 49: 305-313.

Wenger DE, Kendell KR, Miner MR, Trousdale RT. 2004. Acetabular labral tears rarely occur in the absence of bony abnormalities. Clin Orthop Relat Res. 426: 145-150.

Williams P. 1995. Gray's Anatomy, 38th ed. Churchill Livingstone, New York.

Wingstrand H, Wingstrand A, Krantz P. 1990. Intracapsular and atmospheric pressure in the dynamics and stability of the hip. Acta Orthop Scand 61:231-23.

Appendices:

Appendix 1: Femur size in African-American males (n=145): descriptive

Measurements (mm)	African American males			
	Mean	SD	Min	Max
Left femoral anatomical length	468.93	26.49	405	570
Left femoral greater trochanteric length	447.30	24.66	376	512
Left maximum femoral neck length	99.94	5.87	80	118
Left minimum femoral neck length	88.60	6.84	56	106
Left femoral neck shaft angle	127.74	5.58	110	142
Left femoral head diameter	47.90	2.71	38	56
Left femoral neck diameter	33.07	3.14	22	53
Left femoral torsion top	60.46	8.12	43	85
Left femoral torsion bottom	13.07	6.74	0	35
Right femoral anatomical length	468.19	25.58	411	537
Right femoral greater trochanteric length	447.91	26.72	392	579
Right maximum femoral neck length	99.93	5.90	86	118
Right minimum femoral neck length	88.52	6.59	70	108
Right femoral neck shaft angle	129.52	5.53	112	145
Right femoral head diameter	48.34	2.64	39	56
Right femoral neck diameter	33.10	2.69	26	41
Right femoral head torsion top	62.09	7.98	40	82
Right femoral head torsion bottom	14.78	7.85	2	76

Appendix 2: Femur size in African-American females (n=111): descriptive

Measurements (mm)	African American females			
	Mean	SD	Min	Max
Left femoral anatomical length	434.08	24.73	360	482
Left femoral greater trochanteric length	411.97	23.39	345	459
Left maximum femoral neck length	89.23	6.37	78	128
Left minimum femoral neck length	77.42	7.73	64	131
Left femoral neck shaft angle	128.40	8.46	70	147
Left femoral head diameter	41.87	2.65	36	50
Left femoral neck diameter	28.62	2.18	24	34
Left femoral torsion top	53.11	6.48	37	68
Left femoral torsion bottom	11.55	4.87	0	25
Right femoral anatomical length	433.82	23.93	375	495
Right femoral greater trochanteric length	411.86	22.72	356	470
Right maximum femoral neck length	88.93	5.38	78	102
Right minimum femoral neck length	76.50	5.99	60	92
Right femoral neck shaft angle	131.34	6.69	114	148
Right femoral head diameter	41.95	2.64	37	50
Right femoral neck diameter	28.87	2.13	24	34
Right femoral head torsion top	53.63	6.85	38	69
Right femoral head torsion bottom	12.04	5.18	0	26

Appendix 3: Femur size in European- American males (n=177): descriptive

Measurements (mm)	European American males			
	Mean	SD	Min	Max
Left femoral anatomical length	456.51	28.68	393	564
Left femoral greater trochanteric length	435.48	25.47	379	515
Left maximum femoral neck length	100.44	6.52	84	119
Left minimum femoral neck length	91.98	6.50	72	111
Left femoral neck shaft angle	126.20	6.36	109	142
Left femoral head diameter	48.28	2.96	42	56
Left femoral neck diameter	34.33	3.70	27	58
Left femoral torsion top	58.49	7.30	42	75
Left femoral torsion bottom	11.22	5.95	0	29
Right femoral anatomical length	454.56	27.73	386	544
Right femoral greater trochanteric length	433.99	25.37	380	509
Right maximum femoral neck length	100.18	6.54	83	121
Right minimum femoral neck length	91.36	6.55	69	110
Right femoral neck shaft angle	128.15	6.68	106	146
Right femoral head diameter	48.41	2.85	42	56
Right femoral neck diameter	34.08	2.73	27	41
Right femoral head torsion top	59.47	7.73	43	79
Right femoral head torsion bottom	11.66	5.63	0	26

Appendix 4: Femur size in European- American females (n=91): descriptive

Measurement (mm)	European American females			
	Mean	SD	Min	Max
Left femoral anatomical length	417.29	23.48	355	477
Left femoral greater trochanteric length	397.40	24.45	336	473
Left maximum femoral neck length	88.80	5.50	79	104
Left minimum femoral neck length	79.65	6.14	67	94
Left femoral neck shaft angle	126.04	6.23	109	142
Left femoral head diameter	42.13	2.25	36	47
Left femoral neck diameter	29.34	2.01	25	33
Left femoral torsion top	51.16	6.91	38	69
Left femoral torsion bottom	10.10	5.11	0	24
Right femoral anatomical length	416.62	23.07	354	469
Right femoral greater trochanteric length	396.05	22.27	331	442
Right maximum femoral neck length	88.52	5.32	79	102
Right minimum femoral neck length	79.76	5.92	64	94
Right femoral neck shaft angle	128.36	7.44	102	148
Right femoral head diameter	42.29	2.15	37	47
Right femoral neck diameter	29.56	1.92	25	34
Right femoral head torsion top	51.95	6.15	40	67
Right femoral head torsion bottom	10.48	4.57	0	21

Appendix 5: Femur size in African-American and European-American males: T- test

Measurements (mm)	African American males n=145		European American males n=177		P value
	Mean	SD	Mean	SD	
Left femoral anatomical length	468.93	26.49	456.51	28.68	**p<0.001**
Left femoral greater trochanteric length	447.30	24.66	435.48	25.47	**p<0.001**
Left maximum femoral neck length	99.94	5.87	100.44	6.52	0.468
Left minimum femoral neck length	88.60	6.84	91.98	6.50	**p<0.001**
Left femoral neck shaft angle	127.74	5.58	126.20	6.36	**0.021**
Left femoral head diameter	47.90	2.71	48.28	2.96	0.240
Left femoral neck diameter	33.07	3.14	34.33	3.70	**P=0.001**
Left femoral torsion top	60.46	8.12	58.49	7.30	**0.024**
Left femoral torsion bottom	13.07	6.74	11.22	5.95	**0.011**
Right femoral anatomical length	468.19	25.58	454.56	27.73	**p<0.001**
Right femoral greater trochanteric length	447.91	26.72	433.99	25.37	**p<0.001**
Right maximum femoral neck length	99.93	5.90	100.18	6.54	0.719
Right minimum femoral neck length	88.52	6.59	91.36	6.55	**p<0.001**
Right femoral neck shaft angle	129.52	5.53	128.15	6.68	**0.045**
Right femoral head diameter	48.34	2.64	48.41	2.85	0.840
Right femoral neck diameter	33.10	2.69	34.08	2.73	**P=0.001**
Right femoral head torsion top	62.09	7.98	59.47	7.73	**0.003**
Right femoral head torsion bottom	14.78	7.85	11.66	5.63	**p<0.001**
Left femoral shaft bowing angle	159.39	2.09	157.97	1.90	**p<0.001**
Right femoral shaft bowing angle	158.71	2.01	157.29	2.04	**p<0.001**

*Significant p<0.05

Appendix 6: Femur size in African-American and European-American females: T-test

Measurements (mm)	AfAmF n=111		EuAmF n=91		P value
	Mean	SD	Mean	SD	
Left femoral anatomical length	434.08	24.73	417.29	23.48	p<0.001
Left femoral greater trochanteric length	411.97	23.39	397.40	24.45	p<0.001
Left maximum femoral neck length	89.23	6.37	88.80	5.50	0.614
Left minimum femoral neck length	77.42	7.73	79.65	6.14	0.024
Left femoral neck shaft angle	128.40	8.46	126.04	6.23	0.024
Left femoral head diameter	41.87	2.65	42.13	2.25	0.455
Left femoral neck diameter	28.62	2.18	29.34	2.01	0.016
Left femoral torsion top	53.11	6.48	51.16	6.91	0.042
Left femoral torsion bottom	11.55	4.87	10.10	5.11	0.043
Right femoral anatomical length	433.82	23.93	416.62	23.07	p<0.001
Right femoral greater trochanteric length	411.86	22.72	396.05	22.27	p<0.001
Right maximum femoral neck length	88.93	5.38	88.52	5.32	0.587
Right minimum femoral neck length	76.50	5.99	79.76	5.92	p<0.001
Right femoral neck shaft angle	131.34	6.69	128.36	7.44	0.003
Right femoral head diameter	41.95	2.64	42.29	2.15	0.315
Right femoral neck diameter	28.87	2.13	29.56	1.92	0.017
Right femoral head torsion top	53.63	6.85	51.95	6.15	0.067
Right femoral head torsion bottom	12.04	5.18	10.48	4.57	0.025
Left femoral shaft bowing angle	159.68	2.01	157.95	2.25	p<0.001
Right femoral shaft bowing angle	159.45	1.87	157.68	2.13	p<0.001

*Significant p<0.05

Appendix 7: Femur size in African-American females and African-American males: T-test

Measurements (mm)	AfAmF n=111		AfAmM n=145		P value
	Mean	SD	Mean	SD	
Left femoral anatomical length	434.08	24.73	468.93	26.49	p<0.001
Left femoral greater trochanteric length	411.97	23.39	447.30	24.66	p<0.001
Left maximum femoral neck length	89.23	6.37	99.94	5.87	p<0.001
Left minimum femoral neck length	77.42	7.73	88.60	6.84	p<0.001
Left femoral neck shaft angle	128.40	8.46	127.74	5.58	0.483
Left femoral head diameter	41.87	2.65	47.90	2.71	p<0.001
Left femoral neck diameter	28.62	2.18	33.07	3.14	p<0.001
Left femoral torsion top	53.11	6.48	60.46	8.12	p<0.001
Left femoral torsion bottom	11.55	4.87	13.07	6.74	0.038
Right femoral anatomical length	433.82	23.93	468.19	25.58	p<0.001
Right femoral greater trochanteric length	411.86	22.72	447.91	26.72	p<0.001
Right maximum femoral neck length	88.93	5.38	99.93	5.90	p<0.001
Right minimum femoral neck length	76.50	5.99	88.52	6.59	p<0.001
Right femoral neck shaft angle	131.34	6.69	129.52	5.53	0.021
Right femoral head diameter	41.95	2.64	48.34	2.64	p<0.001
Right femoral neck diameter	28.87	2.13	33.10	2.69	p<0.001
Right femoral head torsion top	53.63	6.85	62.09	7.98	p<0.001
Right femoral head torsion bottom	12.04	5.18	14.78	7.85	P=0.001
Left femoral shaft bowing angle	159.68	2.01	159.39	2.09	0.262
Right femoral shaft bowing angle	159.45	1.87	158.71	2.01	0.003

*Significant p<0.05

Appendix 8: Femoral size in European-American females and European-American males: T-test

Measurements (mm)	EuAmF n=91		EuAmM n=177		P value
	Mean	SD	Mean	SD	
Left femoral anatomical length	417.29	23.48	456.51	28.68	p<0.001
Left femoral greater trochanteric length	397.40	24.45	435.48	25.47	p<0.001
Left maximum femoral neck length	88.80	5.50	100.44	6.52	p<0.001
Left minimum femoral neck length	79.65	6.14	91.98	6.50	p<0.001
Left femoral neck shaft angle	126.04	6.23	126.20	6.36	0.850
Left femoral head diameter	42.13	2.25	48.28	2.96	p<0.001
Left femoral neck diameter	29.34	2.01	34.33	3.70	p<0.001
Left femoral torsion top	51.16	6.91	58.49	7.30	p<0.001
Left femoral torsion bottom	10.10	5.11	11.22	5.95	0.111
Right femoral anatomical length	416.62	23.07	454.56	27.73	p<0.001
Right femoral greater trochanteric length	396.05	22.27	433.99	25.37	p<0.001
Right maximum femoral neck length	88.52	5.32	100.18	6.54	p<0.001
Right minimum femoral neck length	79.76	5.92	91.36	6.55	p<0.001
Right femoral neck shaft angle	128.36	7.44	128.15	6.68	0.816
Right femoral head diameter	42.29	2.15	48.41	2.85	p<0.001
Right femoral neck diameter	29.56	1.92	34.08	2.73	p<0.001
Right femoral head torsion top	51.95	6.15	59.47	7.73	p<0.001
Right femoral head torsion bottom	10.48	4.57	11.66	5.63	0.067
Left femoral shaft bowing angle	157.95	2.25	157.97	1.90	0.947
Right femoral shaft bowing angle	157.68	2.13	157.29	2.04	0.146

*Significant p<0.05

Appendix 9: Pelvic size in African-American males (n=115): descriptive

Measurements (mm)	African American males			
	Mean	SD	Min	Max
Posterior-superior iliac spine width	72.49	7.71	54	91
Sciatic notch width	130.44	7.17	115.85	151.27
Spine width	92.33	8.14	74.95	120.67
Ischial tuberosity width	108.71	10.73	82.14	133.59
Anterior superior iliac spine width	219.66	16.37	181.09	259.29
Acetabular depth width	143.32	7.46	127.40	163.60
Superior acetabular width	181.79	9.19	162.90	206.76
Right-ASIS, Right-PSIS	150.56	7.83	128.66	169.48
Left- ASIS, Left-PSIS	149.10	7.78	119.31	167.93
Right horizontal acetabular diameter	53.79	2.91	46.25	60.32
Left horizontal acetabular diameter	53.58	2.99	46.06	62.95
Right vertical acetabular diameter	56.79	2.67	49.90	67.17
Left vertical acetabular diameter	56.38	2.99	50.87	69.91
Pelvic width	259.30	16.53	209	294
Pelvic height	207.21	10.10	189	230
Right acetabular depth	23.31	1.90	19.46	30
Left acetabular depth	23.47	1.78	19.41	28.81
L-Acetabular inclanation angle	65.84	4.91	54.71	75.43
R-Acetabular inclanation angle	65.40	5.03	52.50	77.62
R-Acetabular version angle	49.85	4.21	35.08	59.23
L-Acetabular version angle	46.15	4.66	34.24	59
Sacral inclanation angle	48.01	9.75	20.56	72.07

Appendix 10: Pelvis size in African-American females (n=88): descriptive

Measurements (mm)	African American females			
	Mean	SD	Min	Max
Posterior-superior iliac spine width	81.32	9.93	61	109
Sciatic notch width	134.56	9.03	112.35	155.90
Spine width	109.43	10.4	80.89	132.73
Ischial tuberosity width	127.75	14.18	93.56	178.74
Anterior superior iliac spine width	212.52	18.61	159.63	264.12
Acetabular depth width	147.03	10.36	121.12	170.70
Superior acetabular width	178.12	10.76	152.59	199.80
Right-ASIS, Right-PSIS	144.59	9.40	125.02	165.53
Left- ASIS, Left-PSIS	143,38	9.23	122.50	163.69
Right horizontal acetabular diameter	48.50	3.06	42.01	56.11
Left horizontal acetabular diameter	48.20	2.85	41.19	56.03
Right vertical acetabular diameter	50.63	3.10	44.04	58.49
Left vertical acetabular diameter	50.52	3.04	43.58	58.09
Pelvic width	251.27	18.05	209	289
Pelvic height	191.45	11.22	167	227
Right acetabular depth	21.55	2.07	17.85	27.25
Left acetabular depth	21.55	1.89	18.11	27.36
L-Acetabular inclanation angle	72.19	5.86	55.62	84.14
R-Acetabular inclanation angle	73.07	5.50	56.89	84.23
R-Acetabular version angle	50.26	4.32	38.42	61.59
L-Acetabular version angle	47.96	4.66	36.74	59.85
Sacral inclanation angle	48.89	10.97	23.57	69.71

Appendix 11: Pelvis size in European-American males (n=140): descriptive

Measurements (mm)	European American males			
	Mean	SD	Min	Max
Posterior-superior iliac spine width	78.36	8.80	60	105
Sciatic notch width	139.52	8.80	121.21	159.46
Spine width	96.80	8.72	75.89	126.72
Ischial tuberosity width	116.50	11.17	90.86	148.70
Anterior superior iliac spine width	235.28	18.65	182.61	273.02
Acetabular depth width	150.75	9.57	121.18	176.97
Superior acetabular width	190.58	10.90	158.25	219.63
Right-ASIS, Right-PSIS	157.08	8.83	137.84	175.12
Left- ASIS, Left-PSIS	156.27	8.85	135.54	177.90
Right horizontal acetabular diameter	54.60	3.39	46.61	65.87
Left horizontal acetabular diameter	54.47	3.36	46.33	66.48
Right vertical acetabular diameter	56.46	3.30	47.44	66.92
Left vertical acetabular diameter	56.15	3.45	47.37	68.17
Pelvic width	278.33	19.11	231	320
Pelvic height	214.29	11.59	189	262
Right acetabular depth	23.42	2.02	19.07	29.39
Left acetabular depth	23.86	2.17	18.53	30.28
L-Acetabular inclanation angle	65.37	5.10	53.81	77.19
R-Acetabular inclanation angle	65.17	5.41	51.34	81.31
R-Acetabular version angle	49.80	3.97	40.86	62.75
L-Acetabular version angle	46.27	4.28	34.35	61.59
Sacral inclanation angle	50.29	10.04	27.41	78.32

Appendix 12: Pelvis size in European-American females (n=73): descriptive

Measurements (mm)	European American females			
	Mean	SD	Min	Max
Posterior-superior iliac spine width	82.67	8.75	64	106
Sciatic notch width	142.02	8.34	124.23	161.96
Spine width	111.68	9.92	89.56	139.75
Ischial tuberosity width	129.57	13.92	89.93	185.22
Anterior superior iliac spine width	226.80	20.05	185.67	264.10
Acetabular depth width	153.75	9.09	137.80	173.15
Superior acetabular width	185.46	10.09	165.94	209.17
Right-ASIS, Right-PSIS	151.57	8.53	132.58	167.01
Left- ASIS, Left-PSIS	150.95	8.49	129.77	168.19
Right horizontal acetabular diameter	48.67	2.61	43.35	56.98
Left horizontal acetabular diameter	48.14	2.85	36.73	54.35
Right vertical acetabular diameter	50.65	2.58	44.74	57.48
Left vertical acetabular diameter	50.34	2.33	45.27	55.61
Pelvic width	272.19	18.68	229	320
Pelvic height	195.96	9.19	173	216
Right acetabular depth	21.02	1.96	17.16	26.65
Left acetabular depth	21.02	2.00	16.59	26.04
L-Acetabular inclanation angle	69.81	5.72	58.71	81.32
R-Acetabular inclanation angle	70.55	5.99	55.60	83.81
R-Acetabular version angle	48.68	4.88	36.32	57.98
L-Acetabular version angle	46.20	4.99	33.79	55.00
Sacral inclanation angle	51.10	10.37	22.22	78.48

Appendix 13: Pelvis size in African-American and European-American males: T-test

Measurements (mm)	AfAmM n=115		EuAmM n=140		P value
	Mean	SD	Mean	SD	
Posterior-superior iliac spine width	72.49	7.71	78.36	8.80	p<0.001
Sciatic notch width	130.44	7.17	139.52	8.80	p<0.001
Spine width	92.33	8.14	96.80	8.72	p<0.001
Ischial tuberosity width	108.71	10.73	116.50	11.17	p<0.001
Anterior superior iliac spine width	219.66	16.37	235.28	18.65	p<0.001
Acetabular depth width	143.32	7.46	150.75	9.57	p<0.001
Superior acetabular width	181.79	9.19	190.58	10.90	p<0.001
Right-ASIS, Right-PSIS	150.56	7.83	157.08	8.83	p<0.001
Left- ASIS, Left-PSIS	149.10	7.78	156.27	8.85	p<0.001
Right horizontal acetabular diameter	53.79	2.91	54.60	3.39	0.042
Left horizontal acetabular diameter	53.58	2.99	54.47	3.36	0.026
Right vertical acetabular diameter	56.79	2.67	56.46	3.30	0.383
Left vertical acetabular diameter	56.38	2.99	56.15	3.45	0.559
Pelvic width	259.30	16.53	278.33	19.11	p<0.001
Pelvic height	207.21	10.10	214.29	11.59	p<0.001
Right acetabular depth	23.31	1.90	23.42	2.02	0.641
Left acetabular depth	23.47	1.78	23.86	2.17	0.110
L-Acetabular inclanation angle	65.84	4.91	65.37	5.10	0.460
R-Acetabular inclanation angle	65.40	5.03	65.17	5.41	0.727
R-Acetabular version angle	49.85	4.21	49.80	3.97	0.923
L-Acetabular version angle	46.15	4.66	46.27	4.28	0.842
Sacral inclanation angle	48.01	9.75	50.29	10.04	0.067

*Significant p<0.05

Appendix 14: Pelvis size in African-American and European-American females: T-test

Measurements (mm)	AfAmF n=88		EuAmF n=73		P value
	Mean	SD	Mean	SD	
Posterior-superior iliac spine width	81.32	9.93	82.67	8.75	0.347
Sciatic notch width	134.56	9.03	142.02	8.34	p<0.001
Spine width	109.43	10.4	111.68	9.92	0.165
Ischial tuberosity width	127.75	14.18	129.57	13.92	0.413
Anterior superior iliac spine width	212.52	18.61	226.80	20.05	p<0.001
Acetabular depth width	147.03	10.36	153.75	9.09	p<0.001
Superior acetabular width	178.12	10.76	185.46	10.09	p<0.001
Right-ASIS, Right-PSIS	144.59	9.40	151.57	8.53	p<0.001
Left- ASIS, Left-PSIS	143,38	9.23	150.95	8.49	p<0.001
Right horizontal acetabular diameter	48.50	3.06	48.67	2.61	0.717
Left horizontal acetabular diameter	48.20	2.85	48.14	2.85	0.891
Right vertical acetabular diameter	50.63	3.10	50.65	2.58	0.958
Left vertical acetabular diameter	50.52	3.04	50.34	2.33	0.682
Pelvic width	251.27	18.05	272.19	18.68	p<0.001
Pelvic height	191.45	11.22	195.96	9.19	0.006
Right acetabular depth	21.55	2.07	21.02	1.96	0.097
Left acetabular depth	21.55	1.89	21.02	2.00	0.090
L-Acetabular inclanation angle	72.19	5.86	69.81	5.72	0.010
R-Acetabular inclanation angle	73.07	5.50	70.55	5.99	0.007
R-Acetabular version angle	50.26	4.32	48.68	4.88	0.033
L-Acetabular version angle	47.96	4.66	46.20	4.99	0.023
Sacral inclanation angle	48.89	10.97	51.10	10.37	0.192

*Significant p<0.05

Appendix 15: Pelvis size in European-American females and European-American males: T-test

Measurements (mm)	EuAmF n=73		EuAmM n=140		P value
	Mean	SD	Mean	SD	
Posterior-superior iliac spine width	82.67	8.75	78.36	8.80	P=0.001
Sciatic notch width	142.02	8.34	139.52	8.80	0.044
Spine width	111.68	9.92	96.80	8.72	p<0.001
Ischial tuberosity width	129.57	13.92	116.50	11.17	p<0.001
Anterior superior iliac spine width	226.80	20.05	235.28	18.65	0.003
Acetabular depth width	153.75	9.09	150.75	9.57	0.026
Superior acetabular width	185.46	10.09	190.58	10.90	P=0.001
Right-ASIS, Right-PSIS	151.57	8.53	157.08	8.83	p<0.001
Left- ASIS, Left-PSIS	150.95	8.49	156.27	8.85	p<0.001
Right horizontal acetabular diameter	48.67	2.61	54.60	3.39	p<0.001
Left horizontal acetabular diameter	48.14	2.85	54.47	3.36	p<0.001
Right vertical acetabular diameter	50.65	2.58	56.46	3.30	p<0.001
Left vertical acetabular diameter	50.34	2.33	56.15	3.45	p<0.001
Pelvic width	272.19	18.68	278.33	19.11	0.026
Pelvic height	195.96	9.19	214.29	11.59	p<0.001
Right acetabular depth	21.02	1.96	23.42	2.02	p<0.001
Left acetabular depth	21.02	2.00	23.86	2.17	p<0.001
L-Acetabular inclanation angle	69.81	5.72	65.37	5.10	p<0.001
R-Acetabular inclanation angle	70.55	5.99	65.17	5.41	p<0.001
R-Acetabular version angle	48.68	4.88	49.80	3.97	0.093
L-Acetabular version angle	46.20	4.99	46.27	4.28	0.919
Sacral inclanation angle	51.10	10.37	50.29	10.04	0.586

*Significant p<0.05

Appendix 16: Pelvis size in African-American females and African-American males: T-test.

Measurements (mm)	AfAmF n=88		AfAmM n=115		P value
	Mean	SD	Mean	SD	
Posterior-superior iliac spine width	81.32	9.93	72.49	7.71	p<0.001
Sciatic notch width	134.56	9.03	130.44	7.17	P=0.001
Spine width	109.43	10.4	92.33	8.14	p<0.001
Ischial tuberosity width	127.75	14.18	108.71	10.73	p<0.001
Anterior superior iliac spine width	212.52	18.61	219.66	16.37	0.005
Acetabular depth width	147.03	10.36	143.32	7.46	0.005
Superior acetabular width	178.12	10.76	181.79	9.19	0.011
Right-ASIS, Right-PSIS	144.59	9.40	150.56	7.83	p<0.001
Left- ASIS, Left-PSIS	143.38	9.23	149.10	7.78	p<0.001
Right horizontal acetabular diameter	48.50	3.06	53.79	2.91	p<0.001
Left horizontal acetabular diameter	48.20	2.85	53.58	2.99	p<0.001
Right vertical acetabular diameter	50.63	3.10	56.79	2.67	p<0.001
Left vertical acetabular diameter	50.52	3.04	56.38	2.99	p<0.001
Pelvic width	251.27	18.05	259.30	16.53	P=0.001
Pelvic height	191.45	11.22	207.21	10.10	p<0.001
Right acetabular depth	21.55	2.07	23.31	1.90	p<0.001
Left acetabular depth	21.55	1.89	23.47	1.78	p<0.001
L-Acetabular inclanation angle	72.19	5.86	65.84	4.91	p<0.001
R-Acetabular inclanation angle	73.07	5.50	65.40	5.03	p<0.001
R-Acetabular version angle	50.26	4.32	49.85	4.21	0.499
L-Acetabular version angle	47.96	4.66	46.15	4.66	0.007
Sacral inclanation angle	48.89	10.97	48.01	9.75	0.552

*Significant p<0.05

Appendix 17: Femoral metrical/angular measurements in three groups: No lesion, tongue and ditch.

Measurements	Lesions groups						P Value
	No lesion N.114		Tongue N.133		Ditch N.120		
	Mean	SD	Mean	SD	Mean	SD	
Femoral neck shaft angle	127.3	5.10	127.5	6.20	129.7	5.88	**0.002**
Femoral anatomical length	440.7	29.05	447.7	31.85	453.9	28.77	**0.004**
Greater trochanteric length	420.6	27.24	426.6	32	431	29	**0.015**
Maximum femoral neck length	93.3	7.21	96.6	8.32	96.4	7.70	**0.002**
Minimum femoral neck length	82.78	7.66	87.3	8.51	85.2	8.67	**p<0.001**
Head diameter	45.3	3.88	45.9	4.07	45.7	4	0.442
Neck diameter	31.4	3.15	32	3.73	31.8	3.16	0.366
Femoral torsion top	57.9	7.78	56.7	7.92	56.6	7.47	0.321
Femoral torsion bottom	12.8	5.54	11.3	5.56	11.3	4.97	**0.047**
Femoral shaft bowing angle	158.2	2.07	158.1	1.99	158.5	2.13	0.333

The femur of the ditch group is characterized by greater neck shaft angle, greater femoral and trochanteric length. Both the femur of the tongue and the ditch group manifest a greater neck length and reduced torsion.

Appendix 18: A possible relationship between pelvis metrical/angular characteristic and FHNL.

The pelvis of the tongue and ditch groups manifest a greater horizontal acetabular diameter (tongue 52.6 ± 4.14 and ditch 51.9 ± 3.92 vs. no lesion 51 ± 4.20); a greater sacral inclination angle (tongue 49.1 ± 10.20, ditch 51.1 ± 9.96 and no lesion 47.8 ± 10.93), and greater acetabular depth (tongue 22.6 ± 2.36, ditch 22.9 ± 2.20 and no lesion 21.8 ± 1.99).

Pelvic metrical/angular measurements in two FHNL groups and control: Anova.

Measurements	Lesions groups. (mm)						P Value
	No lesion N.115		Tongue N.133		Ditch N.120		
	Mean	SD	Mean	SD	Mean	SD	
Posterior superior iliac spine width	78.4	9.62	77.4	9.63	78.76	9.49	0.529
Schiatic notch width	135.5	8.95	136.5	9.51	137.1	10.39	0.440
Ischial spine width	101.3	12.29	100.3	11.86	100.7	11.77	0.802
Ischial tuberosity width	117.2	12.39	119.2	15.20	121.1	14.27	0.110
ASIS width	223.2	19.54	226.2	20.7	224.6	20.55	0.509
Acetabular depth width	148.4	9.11	148.2	9.60	149.4	11.19	0.586
Superior acetabular width	183.2	10.48	185.5	11.18	185.3	12.84	0.240
ASIS PSIS width	150.5	10.10	152.3	9.80	152.8	9.82	0.181
Horizontal acetabular diameter	51	4.20	52.6	4.14	51.9	3.92	**0.011**
Vertical acetabular diameter	54.1	4.58	54.3	3.83	54.1	4.25	0.933
Acetabular inclination angle	67.9	4.86	67.3	6.65	67.7	6.99	0.693
Acetabular version angle	48.9	4.30	49.6	4.38	50.2	4.02	0.067
Sacral inclination angle	47.8	10.93	49.1	10.20	51.1	9.96	**0.043**
Pelvic width	264	20.14	268.7	22.39	266.5	21.06	0.216
Pelvic height	202	14.64	205.8	13.89	204.6	13.99	0.097
Acetabular depth	21.8	1.99	22.6	2.36	22.9	2.20	**0.001**

Appendix 19. Interaction between femoral size parameters FHNLs age and sex parameters:

1. No interaction was found between age and sex, age and lesions, sex and lesions, age-sex and lesions in femoral neck shaft angle, femoral neck length minimum, head diameter, neck diameter, femoral torsion top and femoral torsion bottom (P>0.05).

2. Femoral anatomical length was influenced by an interaction between age and lesions (P<0.05).

3. Femoral greater trochanteric length was influenced by an interaction between age and lesions (P<0.05).

4. Maximum femoral neck length was influenced by an interaction between age and lesions (p<0.05).

5. Femoral bowing angle was influenced by an interaction between age and sex (p<0.05).

Interaction between femoral size parameters, FHNLs, age and sex.

Measurements	P Value			
	Age and sex	Age and lesions	Sex and lesions	Age, sex and lesions
Femoral neck shaft angle	0.212	0.802	0.295	0.985
Femoral anatomical length	0.62	**0.021**	0.180	0.170
Greater trochanteric length	0.186	**0.027**	0.089	0.209
Maximum femoral neck length	0.175	**0.017**	0.063	0.361
Minimum femoral neck length	0.950	0.272	0.395	0.060
Head diameter	0.270	0.407	0.397	0.712
Neck diameter	0.513	0.462	0.392	0.306
Femoral torsion top	0.107	0.104	0.378	0.856
Femoral torsion bottom	0.150	0.205	0.291	0.841
Femoral shaft bowing angle	**0.006**	0.238	0.196	0.684

Appendix 20: Anatomical reconstruction of the pelvis.

With the help of strong rubber bands, the innominates were attached to the sacrum (by rearticulating the sacroiliac joint) posteriorly, and anteriorly to each other, at the symphysis pubis area. One rubber was holding the upper part of the pelvis, running just under the ASIS, the second held together the lower parts of the pelvis, the band running at the mid-acetabular level (see figure below). Thin sponges were placed between articulated areas to mimic cartilaginous layers (Howells and Hotelling, 1936; Tague, 1992).

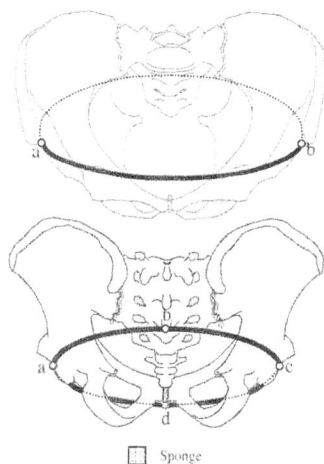

Sponge

Reconstruction of the bony pelvis, anterior view, superior rubber band (top): points a, b: right and left anterior superior iliac spines; posterior view, inferior rubber band (bottom): points a, c: mid acetabular level, point b: sacrum at S4-S5 level, point d: symphysis pubis (adapted from: Peleg et al., 2007).

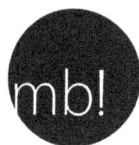

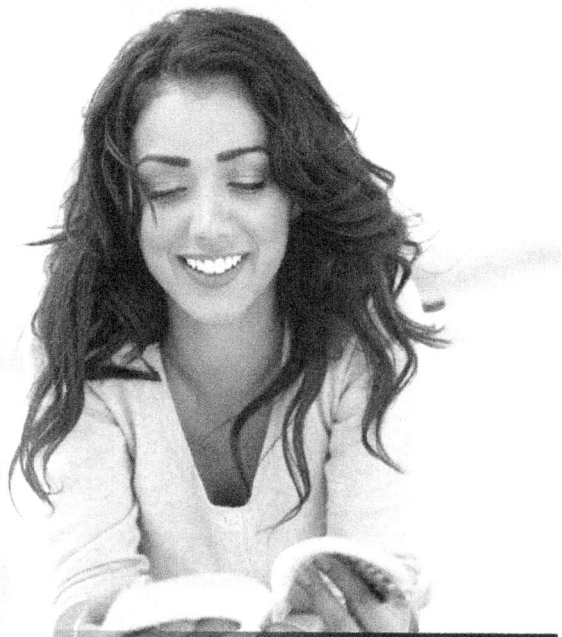

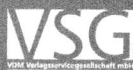

Made in the USA
Coppell, TX
10 April 2021